# DRUG-ELUTING STENTS

Other titles by Christopher J White

Interventional Cardiology: Clinical Applications of New Technologies (1991)
Interventional Cardiology: New Techniques and Strategies for Diagnosis and
Treatment (1994)
Quick Guide to Peripheral Vascular Stenting (2001)
Fifty Cases of Peripheral Vascular Interventions (2001)

# DRUG-ELUTING STENTS

Edited by

**Christopher J White** MD
Chairman, Department of Cardiology
Ochsner Clinic Foundation
New Orleans, LA, USA

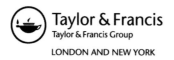
Taylor & Francis
Taylor & Francis Group

LONDON AND NEW YORK

© 2005 Taylor & Francis, an imprint of the Taylor & Francis Group

First published in the United Kingdom in 2005

by Taylor & Francis, an imprint of the Taylor & Francis Group, 2 Park Square, Milton Park, Abingdon, Oxon OX14 4RN

Tel.:       +44 (0) 207 017 6000
Fax.:       +44 (0) 207 017 6699
E-mail:     info.medicine@tandf.co.uk
Website:    http://www.tandf.co.uk/medicine

Although every effort has been made to ensure that all owners of copyright material have been acknowledged in this publication, we would be glad to acknowledge in subsequent reprints or editions any omissions brought to our attention.

Although every effort has been made to ensure that drug doses and other information are presented accurately in this publication, the ultimate responsibility rests with the prescribing physician. Neither the publishers nor the authors can be held responsible for errors or for any consequences arising from the use of information contained herein. For detailed prescribing information or instructions on the use of any product or procedure discussed herein, please consult the prescribing information or instructional material issued by the manufacturer.

A CIP record for this book is available from the British Library.

Library of Congress Cataloging-in-Publication Data

Data available on application

ISBN 1-84214-303-4

Distributed in North and South America by

Taylor & Francis
200 NW Corporate Blvd
Boca Raton, FL 33431, USA
*Within Continental USA*
Tel:      800 272 7737;  Fax: 800 374 3401

*Outside Continental USA*
Tel:      561 994 0555;  Fax: 561 361 6018
E-mail:   orders@crcpress.com

Distributed in the rest of the world by
Thomson Publishing Services
Cheriton House
North Way
Andover, Hampshire SP10 5BE, UK
Tel.:      +44 (0)1264 332424
E-mail:   salesorder.tandf@thomsonpublishingservices.co.uk

Composition by 𝍐 Tek-Art, Croydon. UK

Printed and bound by Cromwell Press Ltd, Trowbridge, Wiltshire

To my mother, Joan Weygandt White, and my father, James Philip White. My mother gave me the gift of unconditional love and taught me the joy of learning. My father was my best friend, my coach, and my first mentor. No son has ever been more fortunate than I.

# Contents

# CONTRIBUTORS

All contributors are from the Department of Cardiology, Ochsner Clinic Foundation, 1514 Jefferson Highway, New Orleans, Louisiana 70121, USA

Ali F Aboufares MD

Salman A Arain MD

Albert W Chan MD

Tyrone J Collins MD

Georges A Feghali MD

J Stephen Jenkins MD

Bahij N Khuri MD

Ali Morshedi-Meibodi MD

Mahesh S Mulumudi MD

Srinivasa P Potluri MD

Stephen R Ramee MD

John P Reilly MD

Jose A Silva MD

Christopher J White MD

# PREFACE

The 'cure' for restenosis has been the Holy Grail of ischemic heart disease since the advent of coronary angioplasty in the late 1970s. Patients were forced to navigate the Scylla and Charybdis of interventional cardiology, having to choose between the 'easier' less morbid angioplasty, and the more 'difficult' but more durable procedure, coronary bypass. The development of stents certainly improved the durability of angioplasty, but in-stent restenosis was a major problem for patients and the physicians who cared for them. The ability to locally deliver drugs on stents that prevent restenosis has been a revolutionary advance in our field. Percutaneous revascularization technology has leaped forward, dramatically altering our clinical practices, with what may be the single most important advance in the history of cardiology.

As with any major advance, there are as many questions raised as answered. We are still in the early stages of our clinical experience with this technology, and there are new delivery platforms and new drugs currently being tested. Despite the continuing advancement, there was a need to collect or collate in a single text, information on drug-eluting stents for coronary disease. My colleagues and I at the Ochsner Clinic Foundation have endeavored to put together a logically organized text that progresses from theory to practice, and addresses pharmacologic, technical, and strategic issues as they relate to the placement of coronary drug-eluting stents. The initial chapters cover the biology of restenosis, alternative methods of treatment, and the pharmacology of anti-restenosis compounds. Later chapters address cost–benefit issues, unapproved indications for drug-eluting stents, and complications related to this technology.

This book is intended for students, cardiology fellows-in-training and practicing clinicians with an interest in Interventional Cardiology and wish to understand the development and use of drug-eluting coronary stent therapy.

# ACKNOWLEDGMENTS

I would like to thank Dr Edward Frohlich, Vice-President of Research at the Ochsner Clinic Foundation, who had the original idea for this book, and my publisher, Jonathan Gregory, whose support and encouragement were much appreciated. I am grateful to Mr Darren Barre for the preparation of the figures and photographs contained in this book. Finally, I must thank my dedicated and hardworking colleagues in the Department of Cardiology at the Ochsner Clinic Foundation, without whom this book would not have been possible.

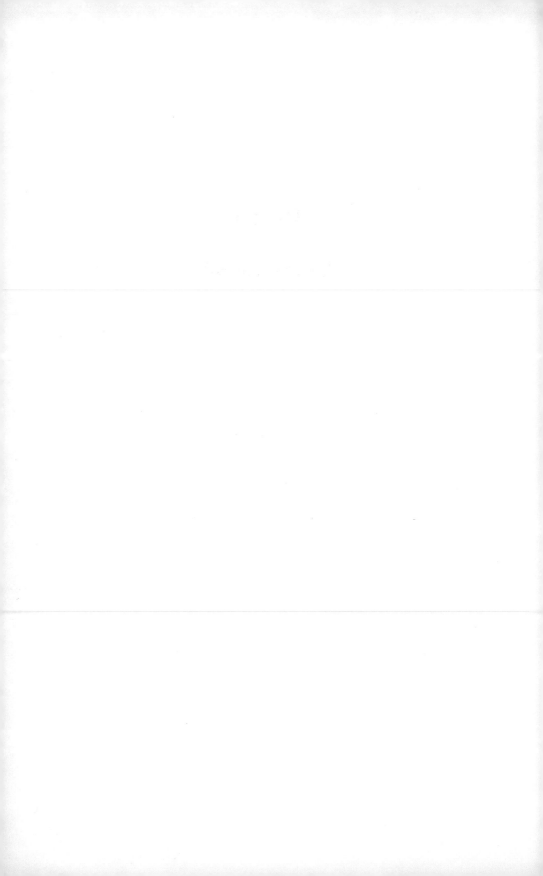

# PART I

# BACKGROUND

# 1. INTRODUCTION AND OVERVIEW

## Christopher J White

## Introduction

The pantheon of coronary revascularization will include milestones such as coronary angiography,[1] coronary revascularization,[2] coronary artery bypass grafting,[3,4] balloon angioplasty,[5] coronary stents,[6–9] adjunctive therapies (high pressure inflation and antiplatelet therapy),[10] and drug-eluting stents.[11–14] It is difficult to argue which of these events was the most important as none of them are singular events but culminations of many smaller pieces of a puzzle which is finally put together. It has been said that innovators stand on the shoulders of those who went before, and that is certainly true in the field of coronary revascularization. The purpose of this book is to collate, in a single volume, the current body of knowledge regarding the clinical experience with drug-eluting stents.

## Drug-eluting stent uncertainty

Drug-eluting stent (DES) indications and useage will evolve over time as more data are collected and larger and more diverse patient populations are studied. The Society of Cardiovascular Angiography and Interventions (SCAI) has published guidelines[15] for practitioners and also surveyed their membership regarding their anticipated DES use (Figures 1.1–1.3). Some of these concerns relate to the most appropriate use of DES. Will there be liability for physicians who do not place DES in selected lesions? Which off-label uses are appropriate and which should be explored before adoption?

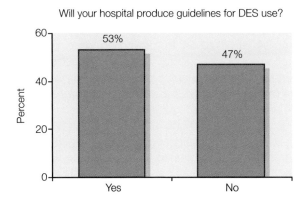

Will your hospital produce guidelines for DES use?

**Figure 1.1:** Society of Cardiovascular Angiography and Interventions (SCAI) survey regarding anticipated hospital guidelines to regulate DES use.

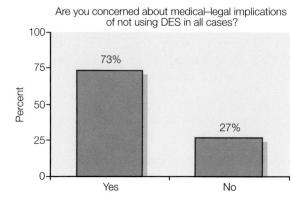

Figure 1.2: Society of Cardiovascular Angiography and Interventions (SCAI) survey regarding anticipated medical–legal liability related to DES useage.

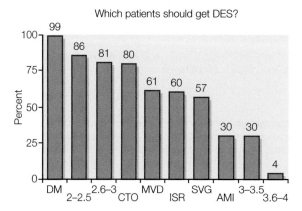

Figure 1.3: Society of Cardiovascular Angiography and Interventions (SCAI) survey regarding which patients or lesions subsets are more likely to be treated with DES. DM, diabetes mellitus; CTO, chronic total occlusion; MVD, multivessel disease; ISR, in-stent restenosis; SVG, saphenous vein graft; AMI, acute myocardial infarction.

## Perspective

In order to put the field of DES into perspective, the initial chapters, Section I, discuss the mechanisms of restenosis, the basic science of antiproliferative coatings, and the development of stent platforms to deliver these agents locally. Section II addresses alternative approaches to preventing or diminishing restenosis. These include pharmacologic agents, mechanical devices, and radiation therapy (brachytherapy). The last chapter in this section reviews the clinical trials comparing bare metal stents (BMS) to percutaneous transluminal coronary angioplasty (PTCA) and heparin-coated stents.

Section III covers the clinical trials, indications, and complications of DES therapy. Section IV discusses patient selection, operator techniques, adjunctive therapies, and treatment strategies to optimize outcomes with DES. The final chapters, Section V, review the cost–benefit analysis for DES, and future directions and applications of DES.

There can be no doubt that the development and implementation of DES in our clinical practices has been a major landmark that will change our approach to the management of coronary artery disease forever. Certainly, more data are required to fully grasp the scope of this benefit and to understand the limitations of this novel therapy. The purpose of this book is to capture the current state of the art in DES therapy, and to put this information into perspective for the reader.

## References

1. Sones FM Jr, Shirey EK. Cine coronary arteriography. Mod Concepts Cardiovasc Dis 1962; 31: 735–38

2. Effler DB, Groves LK, Sones FM Jr et al. Endarterectomy in the treatment of coronary artery disease. J Thorac Cardiovasc Surg 1964; 47: 98–108

3. Fergusson DJ, Shirey EK, Sheldon WC et al. Left internal mammary artery implant – postoperative assessment. Circulation 1968; 37 (4 Suppl): II24–26

4. Favaloro RG. Bilateral internal mammary artery implants. Operative technic – a preliminary report. Cleve Clin Q 1967; 34(1): 61–66

5. Gruntzig A. Transluminal dilatation of coronary-artery stenosis. Lancet 1978; 1(8058): 263

6. Sigwart U, Puel J, Mirkovitch V et al. Intravascular stents to prevent occlusion and restenosis after transluminal angioplasty. N Engl J Med 1987; 316(12): 701–706

7. Roubin GS, King SB 3rd, Douglas JS Jr et al. Intracoronary stenting during percutaneous transluminal coronary angioplasty. Circulation 1990; 81 (3 Suppl): IV92–100

8. Schatz RA, Baim DS, Leon M et al. Clinical experience with the Palmaz–Schatz coronary stent. Initial results of a multicenter study. Circulation 1991; 83(1): 148–61

9. White CJ, Ramee SR, Collins TJ. Elective placement of the Wiktor stent after coronary angioplasty. Am J Cardiol 1994; 74(3): 274–76

10. Colombo A, Hall P, Nakamura S et al. Intracoronary stenting without anticoagulation accomplished with intravascular ultrasound guidance. Circulation 1995; 91(6): 1676–88

11. Sousa JE, Costa MA, Abizaid A et al. Lack of neointimal proliferation after implantation of sirolimus-coated stents in human coronary arteries: a quantitative coronary angiography and three-dimensional intravascular ultrasound study. Circulation 2001; 103(2): 192–95

12. Moses JW, Leon MB, Popma JJ et al. Sirolimus-eluting stents versus standard stents in patients with stenosis in a native coronary artery. N Engl J Med 2003; 349(14): 1315–23

13. Morice MC, Serruys PW, Sousa JE et al. A randomized comparison of a sirolimus-eluting stent with a standard stent for coronary revascularization. N Engl J Med 2002; 346(23): 1773–80

14. Stone GW, Ellis SG, Cox DA et al. A polymer-based, paclitaxel-eluting stent in patients with coronary artery disease. N Engl J Med 2004; 350(3): 221–31

15. Hodgson JM, King SB 3rd, Feldman T et al. SCAI statement on drug-eluting stents: practice and health care delivery implications. Catheter Cardiovasc Interv 2003; 58(3): 397–99.

# 2. Mechanisms of Restenosis Following Percutaneous Coronary Interventions

Salman A Arain and John P Reilly

## Introduction

Percutaneous coronary interventions (PCI) are the most common form of revascularization therapy for atherosclerotic coronary artery disease. Over 1.5 million PCI are performed annually in the USA. The major long-term limitation of PCI is restenosis, the recurrence of the treated blockage. Depending on the modality used and the lesion morphology treated, restenosis affects a substantial number of treated patients. The risk for restenosis is highest in patients with acute coronary syndromes, multivessel disease, and diabetes. The cellular and molecular changes that follow coronary intervention have been extensively characterized in animals and in humans.[1,2] This chapter will describe what is currently known about the pathophysiology of restenosis associated with PCI. This continues to be an active area of research, focused on the identification of effective strategies to prevent or eliminate restenosis.

## Pathophysiology of balloon angioplasty

During balloon inflation in an atherosclerotic lesion, a combination of plaque displacement and vessel expansion result in lumen enlargement.[3] Overdistention of the artery causes endothelial laceration, disruption of the internal elastic lamina, and tears of the medial layer. Stent placement compounds this acute injury by inflicting deeper tissue trauma. These insults provoke an immediate response by the vessel, which includes thrombosis, release of vasoactive agents, and inflammatory cell recruitment.[4] As the acute response to injury abates, a chronic process of healing ensues, characterized by cell proliferation and remodeling of the vessel wall (Figure 2.1).

Three mechanisms are responsible for the development of restenosis: elastic recoil; neointimal proliferation; and negative remodeling. Balloon dilation is followed by immediate elastic recoil of the vessel wall and hematoma formation.[4] The subsequent inflammatory response promotes organization of the thrombus. Over time the inflammatory reaction alters local cytology, resulting in the recruitment and proliferation of smooth muscle cells and fibroblasts. There is increased synthesis of collagen and extracellular matrix, resulting in the formation of a neointima.[1,4] Injury to the adventitia results in the proliferation of adventitial vasa vasorum, and this further promotes cell proliferation and collagen synthesis. Eventually the

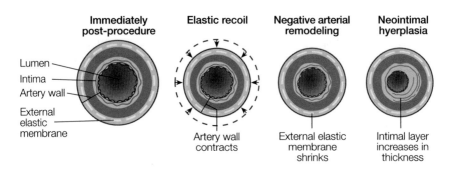

| Immediately post-procedure | Elastic recoil | Negative arterial remodeling | Neointimal hyperplasia |

Lumen
Intima
Artery wall
External elastic membrane

Artery wall contracts

External elastic membrane shrinks

Intimal layer increases in thickness

Figure 2.1: Model of restenosis after percutaneous transluminal coronary angioplasty.

proliferative response reaches a plateau. Maturation of collagen leads to vessel wall shrinkage, a process that has been called negative remodeling.[5] The final lumen diameter is the net effect of cell proliferation, thrombus reorganization, the inflammatory response, and arterial remodeling (Table 2.1).

## Elastic recoil

Balloon dilation results in an acute increase in the vessel lumen diameter. Elastic recoil occurs within seconds to minutes after balloon deflation, reducing the lumen by 40 to 50%. The degree of recoil is related to the elastin content of the internal and external elastic laminae, and is affected very little by balloon size or inflation pressure. Vascular recoil may be defeated by the use of stents, which scaffold the arterial wall.[5]

**Table 2.1. Mechanisms responsible for restenosis following various techniques of coronary revascularization**

| Mechanism | Balloon angioplasty | Cutting balloon | Atherectomy | Laser angioplasty | Bare stent | Drug-eluting stent |
|---|---|---|---|---|---|---|
| Elastic recoil | ++++ | +++ | ++/+++ | ++ | – | – |
| Thrombus formation | ++ | +++ | +++ | +++ | +++ | +++ |
| Neointimal proliferation | ++ | ++ | ++ | ++ | ++++ | +/– |
| Negative remodeling | +++ | +++ | +++ | +++ | – | – |
| Angiographic restenosis | 30–60% | 40–50% | 30–65% | 50–60% | 20–30% | <5 |

## Inflammatory changes

The inflammatory response within the vessel wall following PCI is complex. The cascade of changes that take place at the site of injury can be divided into an early (thrombotic), intermediate (recruitment), and late (proliferative) phases (Figure 2.2).[6]

### Early phase (hours to days): thrombus formation

The early response to endovascular injury is characterized by thrombus formation, and lasts for hours to days following the PCI. PCI-induced vessel trauma is associated with endothelial denudation and dissection of the media, resulting in the exposure of prothrombotic subintimal elements such as collagen, fibronectin, von Willibrand factor, and laminin. Tissue injury and plaque rupture lead to further release of thrombogens such as tissue factor. This results in the rapid, often explosive, activation and aggregation of platelets.[1,7] Within 24 hours there is deposition of fibrin and erythrocytes within the thrombus. Thrombus formation is much more likely to take place following stent deployment. In fact, early vessel occlusion by thrombus may result in catastrophic outcomes following stent placement.

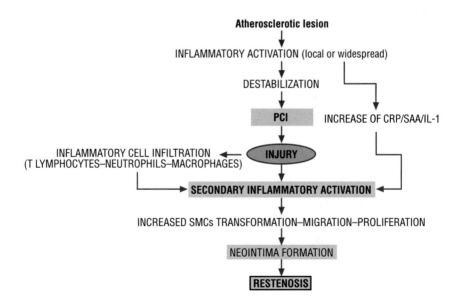

Figure 2.2: The mechanisms by which inflammation is involved before and after percutaneous coronary intervention. (CRP: C-reactive protein; PCI: percutaneous coronary intervention; SAA: serum amyloid A; IL-1: interleukin-1; SMCs: smooth muscle cells.) Reprinted with permission.[6]

### Intermediate phase (3 to 10 days): recruitment

Within days to weeks following PCI, the thrombus begins to organize. Histologically, this stage is characterized by cell recruitment from two sources: the bloodstream and the tunica media. An intense cellular infiltration follows thrombus formation. Chemokines expressed by injured endothelium mediate the influx of hematologic elements such as monocytes (which transform to macrophages as they enter the tissue from the circulating blood), and T-cell lymphocytes.[4] Activated platelets within the thrombus release mitogens such as thromboxane $A_2$, serotonin (5-HT), and platelet-derived growth factor (PDGF).[6] These agents induce endothelial proliferation and migration of vascular smooth muscle cells (VSMCs) from deeper cell layers. Cell proliferation at the site of injury is further promoted by exposure of the cellular elements of the arterial wall to circulating mitogens such as angiotensin II and plasmin.

Data from animal studies suggest that many of the histologic changes following vascular injury are mediated by the activation of early intermediate gene programs. Smooth muscle cell levels of proto-oncogenes such as c-fos, fosB, junB, and junD, rise within days after revascularization. The VSMC phenotype changes from contractile to synthetic, and up to 40% of cells exit the quiescent ($G_0$) phase of the cell cycle.[1] Elaboration of promigratory proteins by activated VSMCs promotes the migration of additional smooth muscle cells from the media and adventitia. This process is inhibited by a healthy endothelium, which produces nitric oxide. Endothelial denudation after angioplasty results in decreased levels of nitric oxide, which removes the inhibitory effect on cell migration and recruitment.[1]

### Late phase (weeks to months): neointimal proliferation

Cell proliferation at the site of injury is accompanied by the synthesis of collagen and the deposition of new extracellular matrix, resulting in the formation of a neointima. Over time, the thrombus is resorbed and eventually replaced by the neointima.[4] Continued cell migration and division increase neointimal volume up to three months after the procedure, with little change after six months. In animal models of stent-induced injury, cell proliferation is most pronounced in the region of the stent strut, suggesting that neointima formation may be an inflammatory (foreign-body) response of the vascular wall.

Mechanisms other than inflammation also contribute to neointimal proliferation. Normalization of shear forces following PCI act to suppress the endothelial production of nitric oxide. This may explain the more sustained neointimal proliferation that occurs following stent placement compared to balloon angioplasty.

## Negative remodeling

Remodeling pertains to temporal changes in arterial size as measured by the area encompassed by the external elastic lamina.[8] This definition does not include neointimal proliferation or plaque volume, which determine residual lumen size without affecting vessel size. Intravascular ultrasound studies in humans have shown that arterial shrinkage accounts for as much as 60% of late lumen loss following balloon angioplasty.[5] The process of negative remodeling may be minimized by stent placement. Restenosis after stenting is associated with little negative remodeling, with late lumen loss due almost exclusively to neointimal hyperplasia.

Several studies have helped to elucidate the mechanisms of negative remodeling in human coronary arteries. Observations from microscopic three-dimensional computed tomography of human coronaries reveal that intense adventitial neovascularization takes place within days following PCI. The amount of vasa vasorum correlates with the percent luminal stenosis.[9] Serial intravascular ultrasound (IVUS) data suggest that thickening and stiffening of the arterial wall may be responsible for changes in the diameter of the artery.[10] It has been proposed that arterial wall shrinkage occurs because of replacement of hyaluronic acid with collagen. Fully remodeled vessels have few actively proliferative cells, and the process has been likened to scar tissue formation in other areas within the body.[11]

# Risk factors for restenosis

A combination of procedural, clinical, and patient characteristics influences the likelihood of restenosis following PCI (Table 2.2). Procedural predictors of

**Table 2.2. Factors associated with restenosis following percutaneous coronary intervention**

| Clinical predictors | Procedural factors |
| --- | --- |
| Acute coronary syndromes | Postprocedural lumen diameter |
| Diabetes mellitus | Percentage residual plaque area |
| Persistent C-reactive protein elevation | Angiographic evidence of thrombus |
| **Lesion characteristics** | **Genetic factors** |
| Long (>10 mm) lesions | Glycoprotein receptor IIIa PIA1/PIA2 |
| Small (<3 mm) vessels | D/D genotype of angiotension-converting |
| Complex lesions | enzyme receptor(?) |
| Chronic total occlusions | 4G/5G promoter of PIA1 |
| Saphenous vein graft | Haptoglobin 2/2 |
| **Stent features** | |
| Length of stent | |
| Thickness of strut metal | |

in-stent restenosis include small vessel size (≤3 mm diameter), greater lesion (stent) length (>10 mm), lesion complexity, and inadequate stent expansion. Some authors have suggested that IVUS imaging should be routinely used to guide stent placement, especially in patients at high risk for restenosis.[12]

Clinical factors that predict in-stent restenosis include the presence of diabetes mellitus, clinical presentation, and perhaps certain genetic factors. Patients with diabetes often have diffuse disease, present with more complex lesions, and demonstrate a greater degree of neointimal hyperplasia following stent placement. Presentation with unstable angina or acute myocardial infarction is associated with higher in-stent restenosis rates. Polymorphisms for the D/D genotype of the angiotensin-converting enzyme inhibitor haptoglobin 2/2 and the glycoprotein receptor IIIa PIA1/PIA2 have also been linked to higher restenosis rates.[13]

## Cutting balloon angioplasty

The cutting balloon is a special device with longitudinally arranged atherotomes on the external surface of the balloon (Figure 2.3). Theoretically, the principle behind the use of the cutting balloon is controlled disruption of atherosclerotic plaque instead of uncontrolled trauma to the vessel wall. The atherotomes would hopefully allow creation of longitudinal fault lines along the luminal surface of the plaque. Subsequent low-pressure balloon inflations would result in axial propagation of the fracture with minimal vessel stretch. Though this mechanism offers an attractive approach to balloon angioplasty, it has met with little success in preventing restenosis. In prospective trials comparing cutting balloon to conventional balloon angioplasty, the rates of angiographic restenosis are identical (Figure 2.4).[14]

## Rotational/directional atherectomy

Prior to the introduction of stent implantation, rotational atherectomy offered an alternative to balloon angioplasty. It was postulated, but never proven, that the use of atherectomy was associated with less vascular injury, and therefore would cause a limited inflammatory and neointimal response. This concept was supported by observations from animal models of coronary stenosis.[15] However, prospective human data, including a recent meta-analysis of 16 trials, have shown that restenosis rates following atherectomy and other ablative therapies for atherosclerotic lesions failed to improve on balloon angioplasty restenosis rates (see Figure 2.4).[14]

Acute lumen gain during atherectomy occurs because of plaque reduction. However, this therapy is associated with a high rate of vascular injury, especially in the presence of eccentric lesions. The extent of arterial wall injury at the time of treatment corresponds directly with the degree of

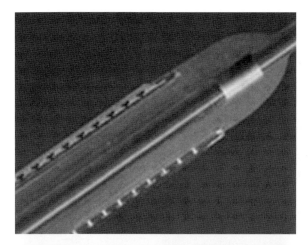

Figure 2.3: (a) Cutting balloon: a balloon with microblades which score the plaque and relax it as it is compacted by the balloon;

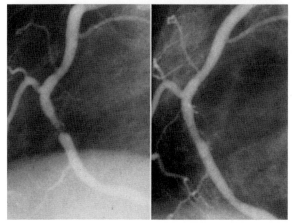

(b) Left panel: baseline stenosis; right panel: after cutting balloon.

subsequent negative remodeling. Longitudinal studies employing IVUS have shown that plaque extension also contributes to late lumen loss following atherectomy.

## Laser angioplasty

Early observations of restenosis following balloon angioplasty showed that lumen diameter at the completion of the procedure was a strong predictor of freedom from restenosis.[16] This led to the concept that lesion debulking, with or without balloon dilation, could increase luminal diameter and improve coronary blood flow while minimizing injury to the vessel wall. It was hypothesized that a laser could be used for plaque ablation and would provide clinical benefit without provoking restenosis. However, this was not borne out by clinical experience.[12] In addition to the unchanged long-term

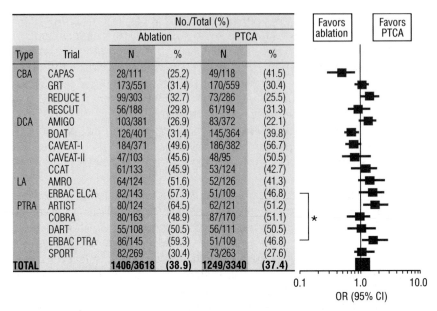

| Type | Trial | No./Total (%) Ablation N | Ablation % | PTCA N | PTCA % |
|------|-------|------|---|------|---|
| CBA | CAPAS | 28/111 | (25.2) | 49/118 | (41.5) |
| | GRT | 173/551 | (31.4) | 170/559 | (30.4) |
| | REDUCE 1 | 99/303 | (32.7) | 73/286 | (25.5) |
| | RESCUT | 56/188 | (29.8) | 61/194 | (31.3) |
| DCA | AMIGO | 103/381 | (26.9) | 83/372 | (22.1) |
| | BOAT | 126/401 | (31.4) | 145/364 | (39.8) |
| | CAVEAT-I | 184/371 | (49.6) | 186/382 | (56.7) |
| | CAVEAT-II | 47/103 | (45.6) | 48/95 | (50.5) |
| | CCAT | 61/133 | (45.9) | 53/124 | (42.7) |
| LA | AMRO | 64/124 | (51.6) | 52/126 | (41.3) |
| | ERBAC ELCA | 82/143 | (57.3) | 51/109 | (46.8) |
| PTRA | ARTIST | 80/124 | (64.5) | 62/121 | (51.2) |
| | COBRA | 80/163 | (48.9) | 87/170 | (51.1) |
| | DART | 55/108 | (50.5) | 56/111 | (50.5) |
| | ERBAC PTRA | 86/145 | (59.3) | 51/109 | (46.8) |
| | SPORT | 82/269 | (30.4) | 73/263 | (27.6) |
| **TOTAL** | | **1406/3618** | **(38.9)** | **1249/3340** | **(37.4)** |

Figure 2.4: Angiographic restenosis rates between 90 and 360 days. There is no advantage for debulking therapy over balloon angioplasty alone. CBA, cutting balloon angioplasty; DCA, directional coronary atherectomy; LA, laser angioplasty; PTRA, percutaneous transluminal rotational atherectomy. * = the ERBAC control groups are identical. Reprinted with permission.[14]

rates of restenosis, early experiences with laser angioplasty were frequently associated with procedural complications such as perforations and dissections.

Laser angioplasty, with or without adjunctive angioplasty, is associated with limited acute luminal gain. The rates of early reduction in lumen size following laser ablation are identical to those following balloon angioplasty (≥40% within 30 days), primarily because of elastic recoil (see Figure 2.4).[14] Rates of late lumen loss are also similar and, in the absence of stent implantation, approach 80%.

## Bare metal stents

Stent placement represents an important and successful approach to restenosis following balloon angioplasty. However, the use of bare metal stents are associated with a 20 to 30% risk of restenosis.[1] As the rates of coronary stent placement increase globally, in-stent restenosis presents a greater challenge.

Stenting resists immediate elastic recoil and therefore eliminates early lumen loss. However, stenting causes more profound trauma to the arterial wall because of strut penetration. Stenting is associated with a greater degree of thrombogenesis because of strut-induced disruption of the subintima and greater release of tissue factor. A negative charge on the stent surface also attracts platelets immediately after deployment. The presence of the stent metal incites a stronger and more sustained inflammatory response because of lipid core exposure and medial trauma. This is confirmed by a greater degree of inflammatory cell infiltration in the region of the struts. Expression of monocyte chemokine (MCP-1) and interleukin-8 is transient following angioplasty, but sustained following stent injury.[4] Animal data suggest that the magnitude of early inflammatory reaction after stent implantation predicts the amount of neointimal proliferation that will follow. In humans, coronary stenting accompanied by strut penetration of the lipid core or medial damage is associated with greater neointimal thickness and higher rates of restenosis.[4]

Animal studies and necroscopy specimen data have demonstrated that the major component of in-stent restenosis is neointimal proliferation. Neointimal thickness increases for up to six months after stent deployment, after which it abates at a variable rate. Initially both macrophages and activated VSMCs can be identified within the neoproliferate. After six months, few actively dividing cells remain. The in-stent tissue at this stage is principally composed of matrix proteoglycans and collagen, with 10% or less being contributed by cells (mostly activated VSMCs).[9] Most proliferative cells are located close to stent struts, which bolsters the idea that neointima formation represents a low-grade reaction to the stent.

## Drug-eluting stents

The introduction of drug-eluting stents has revolutionized PCI. Efficacy data from clinical studies have shown restenosis rates of 5% or lower.[2,16,17] Drug-eluting stents work by inhibiting the multiple biological processes that constitute restenosis. The stent scaffolds the vessel to prevent recoil, while bioactive agents delivered by the stent affect the surrounding tissue and prevent neointimal hyperplasia (Figure 2.5). Stents provide the ideal vehicle for

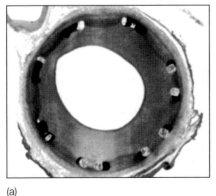
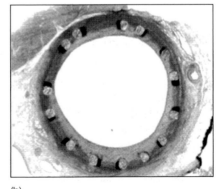

(a)                    (b)

Figure 2.5: Porcine arteries. (a) Control bare metal stent; (b) Sirolimus drug-eluting stent.

drug delivery because their proximity to the site of injury allows higher concentrations of the active agent to be delivered locally without causing systemic effects.

## Conclusion

The major limitation of PCI is restenosis. Several overlapping processes contribute to the development of restenosis, including elastic recoil, thrombus formation, neointimal proliferation, and negative remodeling. The net gain (or loss) in lumen size following revascularization depends on the balance between these components of the vascular response to injury. In addition to hundreds of pharmacologic therapies, many different revascularization techniques have been investigated in an effort to prevent de-novo restenosis. Many of the device therapies were developed under the premise that minimizing trauma to the vessel wall will yield lower restenotic rates. This approach has been largely unsuccessful. Effective treatments have succeeded by counteracting the mechanical and/or biological processes that follow vessel injury.

## References

1. Bauters C, Isner JM. The biology of restenosis. In: Topol EJ, ed. Textbook of Cardiovascular Medicine. Philadelphia: Lippincott-Raven; 1998: pp. 2465–90

2. Holmes DR Jr, Leon MB, Moses JW et al. Analysis of 1-year clinical outcomes in the SIRIUS trial: a randomized trial of a sirolimus-eluting stent versus a standard stent in patients at high risk for coronary restenosis. Circulation 2004; 109(5): 634–40

3. Ahmed JM, Mintz GS, Weissman NJ et al. Mechanism of lumen enlargement during intracoronary stent implantation: an intravascular ultrasound study. Circulation 2000; 102(1): 7–10

4. Farb A, Sangiorgi G, Carter AJ et al. Pathology of acute and chronic coronary stenting in humans. Circulation 1999; 99(1): 44–52

5. Mintz GS, Popma JJ, Pichard AD et al. Arterial remodeling after coronary angioplasty: a serial intravascular ultrasound study. Circulation 1996; 94: 35–43

6. Toutouzas K, Colombo A, Stefanadis C. Inflammation and restenosis after percutaneous coronary interventions. Eur Heart J 2004; 25(19): 1679–87

7. Pakala R, Willerson JT, Benedict CR. Effect of serotonin, thromboxane A2, and specific receptor antagonists on vascular smooth muscle cell proliferation. Circulation 1997; 96(7): 2280–86

8. Schwartz RS, Topol EJ, Serruys PW et al. Artery size, neointima, and remodeling: time for some standards. J Am Coll Cardiol 1998; 32: 2087–94

9. Kwon HM, Sangiorgi G, Ritman EL et al. Adventitial vasa vasorum in balloon-injured coronary arteries: visualization and quantitation by a microscopic three-dimensional computed tomography technique. J Am Coll Cardiol 1998; 32: 2072–79

10. Sangiorgi G, Taylor AJ, Farb A et al. Histopathology of postpercutaneous transluminal coronary angioplasty remodeling in human coronary arteries. Am Heart J 1999; 138 (4 Pt 1): 681–87

11. Moreno PR, Palacios IF, Leon MN et al. Histopathologic comparison of human coronary in-stent and post-balloon angioplasty restenotic tissue. Am J Cardiol 1999; 84(4): 462–66, A9

12. Kasaoka S, Tobis JM, Akiyama T et al. Angiographic and intravascular ultrasound predictors of in-stent restenosis. J Am Coll Cardiol 1998; 32(6): 1630–35

13. Kastrati A, Schomig A, Seyfarth M et al. PIA polymorphism of platelet glycoprotein IIIa and risk of restenosis after coronary stent placement. Circulation 1999; 99(8): 1005–10

14. Bittl JA, Chew DP, Topol EJ et al. Meta-analysis of randomized trials of percutaneous transluminal coronary angioplasty versus atherectomy, cutting balloon atherectomy, or laser angioplasty. J Am Coll Cardiol 2004; 43(6): 936–42

15. McKenna CJ, Wilson SH, Camrud AR et al. Neointimal response following rotational atherectomy compared to balloon angioplasty in a porcine model of coronary in-stent restenosis. Catheter Cardiovasc Diag 1998; 45(3): 332–36

16. Farb A, Weber DK, Kolodgie FD et al. Morphological predictors of restenosis after coronary stenting in humans. Circulation 2002; 105(25): 2974–80

17. Stone GW, Ellis SG, Cox DA et al. One-year clinical results with the slow-release, polymer-based, paclitaxel-eluting TAXUS stent: the TAXUS-IV trial. Circulation 2004; 109(16): 1942–47

18. Grube E, Sonoda S, Ikeno F et al. Six- and twelve-month results from first human experience using everolimus-eluting stents with bioabsorbable polymer. Circulation 2004; 109(18): 2168–71

# 3. Drug-Eluting Stent Platforms: Antiproliferative Drugs and Polymer Coatings

## Albert W Chan

## Introduction

The pathogenesis of restenosis after coronary angioplasty is a complex process and it includes early recoil, thrombus formation, arterial remodeling, and neointimal hyperplasia.[1] Neointimal hyperplasia is the sole mediator of in-stent restenosis and is the result of smooth muscle cell activation, proliferation, and migration, and extracellular matrix synthesis, beginning as early as 48 hours after stent implantation,[2–4] and is predominant within the first 30 days.[5,6] Strategies to inhibit restenosis involve the targeting of one or a combination of these reparative processes (Figure 3.1). Systemic delivery of drugs to reduce restenosis is limited by their systemic toxicity.[7] A controlled, local delivery of antiproliferative agents using a stent platform should increase the drug concentration at the target site while minimizing the systemic effects of the drugs. Various modalities of stent-based drug delivery are being used

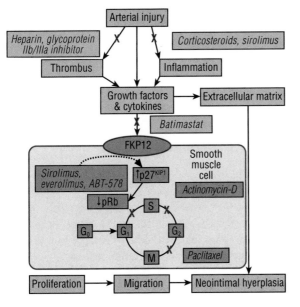

Figure 3.1: Therapeutic targets to prevent in-stent restenosis.

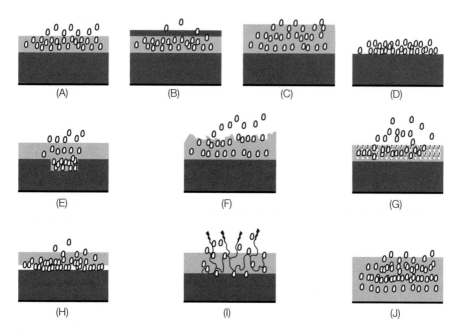

Figure 3.2: Schematic representation of different modalities of drug-eluting stent platforms (black : stent strut; gray : coating; circles : drug). (a) Drug–polymer blend, release by diffusion. (b) Drug diffusion through additional polymer coating. (c) Drug release by swelling of coating. (d) Non-polymer-based drug release. (e) Drug loaded in stent reservoir. (f) Drug release by coating erosion. (g) Drug loaded in nanoporous coating reservoirs. (h) Drug loaded between coatings (coating sandwich). (i) Polymer–drug conjugate cleaved by hydrolysis or enzymic action. (j) Biodegradable polymeric stent. (Reprinted from Sousa JE, Serruys PW, Costa MA. New frontiers in cardiology: drug-eluting stents. Part I. Circulation 2003; 107: 2274–2279, with permission from Lippincott Williams and Wilkins.)

or are under evaluation (Figure 3.2). Indeed, clinical trials have confirmed the efficacy of this strategy in reducing clinical and angiographic restenosis in clinical practice.[8–10] In this chapter, the pharmacology of various antiproliferative agents and the polymer for drug-eluting stent technology will be reviewed.

## Polymer stent coatings

Inorganic stent coatings (e.g. silicon carbide, diamond-like carbon, gold, titanium, nitride oxide alloy) have been used to improve the biocompatibility of metal stents, but these coatings have either neutral effects in humans or some cases may increase restenosis.[11–17] Inorganic coatings cannot incorporate drugs and facilitate a controlled local delivery. Another strategy was to use heparin bonding, which has been shown to reduce thrombogenicity of some indwelling devices.[18,19] However, when tested on various stent platforms (Palmaz–Schatz stent, Wiktor stent, JOSTENT®) in human coronary arteries, heparin bonding did not reduce intimal hyperplasia.[20–22]

Polymers are long chains of repetitive molecular units; when applied to the stent their purpose is to contain the drug and allow its gradual release. Box 3.1 lists the properties of an ideal organic polymer for stent coating. A number of polymers have been tested but one that has been brought to clinical use is the non-erodable poly-*n*-butyl methacrylate and polyethylene vinyl acetate copolymer that has been applied on the Cordis Bx VELOCITY™ stainless steel stent. This polymer is applied as a wet solution on the stent and is dried in a proprietary manner to bind onto the stent metal, resulting in a final thickness of 5 µm. Sirolimus (140 µg/cm$^2$) is attached to the coating in a proprietary manner and the total weight of the drug and polymer is about 500 µg. This stent can be formulated into fast release (<15-day drug release) and slow release (≥28-day drug release) but only the slow-release formulation has been tested in clinical trials.[23] The slow-release coating is formulated by applying a top coating in addition to the base coating. The serum sirolimus level reaches its peak (0.9 ± 0.2 ng/ml) at 1 hour after stent implantation and becomes undetectable (0.4 ng/ml) by 72 hours.[24] The drug is released by diffusion.[24,25]

**Box 3.1 Properties of an ideal polymer for stent coating**

- Low profile for easy deliverability of the stent
- Conform to the artery lumen and shape
- Absolute plasticity to enable stent expansion without disruption of the coating
- Resistant to wearing or tearing within the artery or during stent delivery
- Adequate surface area to deliver the assigned drug dose
- Not to result in hypersensitivity or other local inflammatory reactions and fibrosis within the artery

The Boston Scientific paclitaxel-eluting Express™ stent (PES) uses poly(lactide-co-Σ-caprolactone) copolymer as a vehicle to carry paclitaxel, the dose of which was refined in a series of animal studies. The copolymer remains inert up to 6 months after implantation. Similar to the sirolimus-eluting stent, paclitaxel is distributed to the surrounding arterial tissue under the force of diffusion and convection.[26]

Concerns have been raised with regard to hypersensitivity reactions caused by the polymer coatings,[27] and therefore attempts have been made to build non-polymer-based drug-coated stents. Paclitaxel is one of the few drugs that can be applied directly onto the stent without a polymer matrix. The results of the clinical studies using non-polymer-based paclitaxel delivery have been inconclusive. Cook has sponsored three clinical trials that involved non-polymer-based stents. In the European Evaluation of Paclitaxel-Eluting Stent (ELUTES) study,[28] the V-Flex stents (Cook, Inc.) were loaded with four different doses of paclitaxel (0.2, 0.7, 1.4, and 2.7 µg/mm$^2$) with a proprietary method, and were compared with the bare metal stent. A dose-dependent effect of paclitaxel on intimal proliferation was reported, but the clinical events were not different at 1 year. In the Asian Paclitaxel-Eluting Clinical Trial (ASPECT),[29] the paclitaxel-coated Supra-G stents (Cook, Inc.) also showed suppression of late loss in a dose-dependent manner at 6 months (in-stent late loss 0.29 mm in 3.1 µg/mm$^2$, 0.57 mm in 1.3 µg/mm$^2$, and 1.04 mm in the controls). The Paclitaxel-Eluting Stent for Cytostatic Prevention of Restenosis (PATENCY) using Logic PTX (Cook, Inc.) did not show any difference in restenosis with the paclitaxel coating (2.0 µg/mm$^2$) (Alan Heldman MD, Johns Hopkins University, unpublished data, 2002). In the DELIVER trial,[30] the non-polymer paclitaxel-coated Achieve™ stent (3 µg/mm$^2$ of paclitaxel) was compared with bare Multilink Penta (Guidant) stent and the result showed a non-significant reduction of neointimal hyperplasia in the Achieve™ stent arm, perhaps due to the low restenosis rate with the Penta stent. In summary, these trials suggest an important role of controlled release of the drug over time using a polymer coating.

## Paclitaxel

Paclitaxel can be obtained from the bark of the pacific yew tree (*Taxus brevifolia*) in the north-western USA, and is synthetically manufactured as an antineoplastic drug (Taxol) approved for the treatment of ovarian cancer (Figure 3.3).[31] It inhibits cell proliferation and migration by assembling the tubulin dimers into the non-functional microtubules, leading to the alteration of the cell cytoskeleton structure.[32,33] By inhibiting the depolymerization of

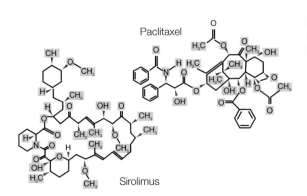

Figure 3.3: Molecular structures of sirolimus and paclitaxel.

the microtubules, the drug further prohibits the activation of protein kinase and transcription factor release.[34,35] The drug is highly lipophilic, resulting in a rapid uptake of the drug across the cell membrane and a prolonged tissue retention time. When given to animals at a plasma level 100 times less than the dose used for anticancer therapy in humans, paclitaxel inhibits vascular smooth muscle cell proliferation and migration after balloon injury.[36] The dose used for local delivery on a stent is 3000 times less than the concentration used for systemic chemotherapy. When impregnated with poly(lactide-co-$\Sigma$-caprolactone) copolymer onto NIR stents (Boston Scientific, Inc.), suppression of neointimal hyperplasia was observed for up to 6 months in porcine coronary arteries.[37]

For clinical studies, the fast-release (FR) paclitaxel-eluting stent (PES) contains $2.04\,\mu g/mm^2$ of paclitaxel (~171 $\mu$g for a 7 cell/15 mm stent), and both the moderate- and the slow-release (MR and SR) stents contain $1.0\,\mu g/mm^2$ (~85 $\mu$g/stent) paclitaxel.[38,39] The TAXUS II trial compared the SR and MR formulations on the NIRx Conformer stent.[39] In this stent, the drug was released with an initial burst phase for 48 hours after implantation followed by a low-level release phase for approximately 10 days. The major difference of the two formulations was that there was 8-fold higher amount of the dose release in MR compared with SR over the first 10 days. Of the total dose, 75% remains sequestered within the MR stent and 90% within the SR stent without any further measurable release of paclitaxel. In an animal model, paclitaxel provides a dose-dependent inhibition of neointimal hyperplasia.[40] The clinical results of the clinical trials (TAXUS I–VI) with this stent will be discussed in the other chapters.

## Sirolimus

Sirolimus (rapamycin) is a macrolide antifungal antibiotic isolated from *Streptomyces hygroscopicus* (see Figure 3.3). It has been approved as an immunosuppressive drug in renal transplantation.[41] By binding to a cytosolic receptor, FK506 binding protein (FKBP12), it increases the cellular cyclin-dependent kinase inhibitor (CDKI) p27$^{kip1}$ levels and inhibits the phosphorylation of retinoblastoma protein (pRb) activity, a critical regulator of vascular smooth muscle cell proliferation (see Figure 3.1).[42] This drug inhibits vascular smooth muscle cell proliferation and migration by arresting the cell cycle at the $G_1/S$ transition.[42–46] The drug is lipophilic and therefore is readily taken up across the cell membrane.[47,48]

Marx and coworkers demonstrated the inhibition of vascular smooth muscle cell proliferation with sirolimus in both human and rat in vitro models through blocking the $G_1/S$ phase.[43,44] Gallo et al further showed that systemic infusion of sirolimus could inhibit restenosis after balloon angioplasty in porcine coronary artery.[42] This suggested that sirolimus could be used to inhibit neointimal hyperplasia after stenting with its antiproliferative property. Semi-quantitative histologic grading of the sirolimus-eluting stents in animal model revealed a significantly lower smooth muscle cell content and a higher fibrin deposition, but similar endothelial contents, when compared with that of bare metal stents.[25,49]

## Everolimus

Everolimus, 40-O-(2-hydroxyethyl)-rapamycin, is an analog of rapamycin and inhibits cellular proliferation using the same pathway as in rapamycin, but the immunosuppressive activity of everolimus is two- to threefold lower than that of sirolimus in vitro.[23] Oral everolimus has been shown to reduce in-stent restenosis in animal models.[23,50] Everolimus- and sirolimus-eluting stents were shown to be equally effective in reducing neointimal proliferation in a porcine coronary model.[51] The Challenge™ stent incorporates the S-Stent platform (Biosensor) which is coated with the low-dose (180 mg/stent) or high-dose (360 mg/stent) everolimus using the biodegradable hydroxyacid polylactic acid polymer. Initial experience in humans with this stent suggested that it was effective in suppressing restenosis.[52,53] It is now undergoing evaluation in large-scale clinical studies (First Use To Underscore Reduction in restenosis with Everolimus: FUTURE III–IV).

## ABT-578

ABT-578, or methyl-rapamycin, is another synthetic analog of rapamycin. It is applied onto Bio*div*Ysio® stent and the initial feasibility study (ENDEAVOR I) was completed, with a 4-month major adverse cardiac events of 2.0%.[54] Subsequent large-scale studies will examine the efficacy of the stent when compared with the approved Cypher stents (ENDEAVOR II–III).

## Tacrolimus

Tacrolimus binds to FKBP12 protein. Different from sirolimus, it does not inhibit smooth muscle cell growth, but inhibits proinflammatory cytokines and T-cell activation.[44] The drug was evaluated for stent-based delivery in de-novo lesions (PRESENT) and in saphenous vein graft lesions (EVIDENT) using the Flexmaster (Jomed) nanoporous ceramic and Jomed PTFE-covered stent platforms respectively, but both studies failed to show a reduction of restenosis with the stents.[55,56]

## Angiopeptin

Angiopeptin has been shown to reduce restenosis by inhibiting tissue response to several growth factors (e.g. platelet-derived growth factor, fibroblast, and insulin-like growth factors). It has been shown to reduce neointimal hyperplasia in animal models when impregnated onto the stent with polymers.[57,58] The long-term outcome of an angiopeptin-eluting Bio*div*Ysio® stent is being examined in the SWAN study.[59]

## C-myc antisense-eluting stent

Systemic gene therapy has been hampered by inefficient uptake of the vector by the target. Local gene delivery using stents is a novel therapeutic approach to reduce restenosis. C-myc is important in the regulation of cell division and cell proliferation. C-myc antisense oligonucleotides may block gene expression via specific complementary deoxyribonucleic acid sequences to small segments of the messenger ribonucleic acid. Target proteins may be cytotoxic, or inhibitory to growth factors, cell differentiation, or proliferation. A randomized clinical study that examined the effectiveness of phosphorothioate-modified oligonucleotide against c-myc did not show any benefit when compared to controls.[60] More recently, a six-ring morpholino backbone c-myc antisense (AVI-4126)-eluting stent using phosphocholine coating was shown to inhibit intimal hyperplasia and allowed re-endothelialization when implanted in a porcine balloon-injury model.[61]

## Anti-inflammatory agents

Restenosis begins with inflammation, followed by proliferation, migration, and extracellular matrix production. Dexamethasone has been applied onto the Bio*divYsio*® stent using phosphocholine coating, and has been studied in the Study of Anti-Restenosis with Bio*divYsio*® Dexamethasone-eluting stent (STRIDE) study.[62] The result of this feasibility study showed a 3% target lesion revascularization at 6 months. A long-term 1000-patient registry (SAFE registry) is to evaluate the 'real-world' outcome of the Dexamet™ stent.

## Pro-healing agents

Endothelial denudation occurs after balloon angioplasty and may promote vascular thrombosis and restenosis. Early re-endothelialization and restoration of endothelial function may abort the restenotic process. Nitric oxide, vascular endothelial growth factor, and 17-β-estradiol, have been loaded onto the stents and data on whether they prevent restenosis are still lacking. Attempts have also been made to attach a monolayer of antibodies to CD34 receptors, which are located on the surface of the circulating endothelial cells.

## Estradiol

Estradiol promotes endothelialization and inhibits smooth muscle cell migration and proliferation.[63] Estradiol-eluting phosphocholine-controlled stents produce 40% reduction in neointimal hyperplasia.[64] The implantation of 17-β-estradiol-eluting Bio*divYsio*® stent has been completed in 30 patients enrolled in the Estrogen And Stents To Eliminate Restenosis (EASTER) trial, and four (13%) patients had angiographic restenosis >50% at follow-up.[65] The Phase II portion of this trial is still ongoing.

## Extracellular matrix modulators

Matrix metalloproteinase (MMP) can degrade collagen and extracellular protein, and hence facilitate smooth muscle cell migration. Batimastat, a non-specific MMP inhibitor, has been shown to reduce late lumen loss by preventing constrictive arterial remodeling in animal models, without any effect on neointimal hyperplasia.[66] Batimastat delivery from phosphocholine-coated stents has been found to reduce neointimal hyperplasia in a swine model.[67] However, further clinical study has been on hold since the lack of efficacy of the batimastat-eluting stent in preventing restenosis was shown in the Batimastat Anti-Restenosis trial Utilizing the Bio*divYsio*® Local Delivery PC-Stent (BRILLIANT-I) study.

## Anti-thrombotic and antiplatelet agents

While platelet aggregation and thrombosis play an important role in vascular injury and restenosis, antiplatelet therapy and anticoagulation, either given systemically or by stent-based delivery, have not been shown to have a significant effect on anti-restenosis therapy. Heparin, glycoprotein IIb/IIIa antagonist, hirudin, and nitric oxide have been applied as a stent coating, but the data of their clinical effectiveness have not yet been demonstrated.[20,68,69]

## References

1. Chan AW, Moliterno DJ. Restenosis: The clinical issues. In Topol EJ, ed. Textbook of Interventional Cardiology. Philadelphia: Saunders; 2003: pp. 415–54

2. Clowes AW, Reidy MA, Clowes MM. Kinetics of cellular proliferation after arterial injury. I. Smooth muscle growth in the absence of endothelium. Lab Invest 1983; 49: 327–33

3. Forrester JS, Fishbein M, Helfant R et al. A paradigm for restenosis based on cell biology: clues for the development of new preventive therapies. J Am Coll Cardiol 1991; 17: 758–69

4. Farb A, Sangiorgi G, Carter AJ et al. Pathology of acute and chronic coronary stenting in humans. Circulation 1999; 99: 44–52

5. Virmani R, Farb A. Pathology of in-stent restenosis. Curr Opin Lipidol 1999; 10: 499–506

6. Nobuyoshi M, Kimura T, Nosaka H et al. Restenosis after successful percutaneous transluminal coronary angioplasty: serial angiographic follow-up of 229 patients. J Am Coll Cardiol 1988; 12: 616–23

7. Lincoff AM, Topol EJ, Ellis SG. Local drug delivery for the prevention of restenosis. Fact, fancy, and future. Circulation 1994; 90: 2070–84

8. Morice MC, Serruys PW, Sousa JE et al. A randomized comparison of a sirolimus-eluting stent with a standard stent for coronary revascularization. N Engl J Med 2002; 346: 1773–80

9. Moses JW, Leon MB, Popma JJ et al. Sirolimus-eluting stents versus standard stents in patients with stenosis in a native coronary artery. N Engl J Med 2003; 349: 1315–23

10. Stone GW, Ellis SG, Cox DA et al. A polymer-based, paclitaxel-eluting stent in patients with coronary artery disease. N Engl J Med 2004; 350: 221–31

11. Heublein B, Pethig K, Elsayed AM. Silicon carbide coating: A semiconducting hybrid design of coronary stents. A feasibility study. J Invasive Cardiol 1998; 10: 255–62

12. Antoniucci D, Bartorelli A, Valenti R et al. Clinical and angiographic outcome after coronary arterial stenting with the carbostent. Am J Cardiol 2000; 85: 821–25

13. Kastrati A, Schomig A, Dirschinger J et al. Increased risk of restenosis after placement of gold-coated stents: results of a randomized trial comparing gold-coated with uncoated steel stents in patients with coronary artery disease. Circulation 2000; 101: 2478–83

14. Edelman ER, Seifert P, Groothuis A et al. Gold-coated NIR stents in porcine coronary arteries. Circulation 2001; 103: 429–34

15. Windecker S, Mayer I, De Pasquale G et al. Stent coating with titanium–nitride-oxide for reduction of neointimal hyperplasia. Circulation 2001; 104: 928–33

16. Hamm C. A multicenter, randomized trial comparing silicon carbide-coated stents with stainless steel stents in acute coronary syndrome (TRUST study). Circulation 2001; 104 (Suppl): II464

17. Herrmann RA, Rybnikar A, Resch A et al. Thrombogenicity of stainless steel coronary stents with a completely gold coated surface. J Am Coll Cardiol 1998; 31: 413A

18. Hoar PF, Wilson RM, Mangano DT et al. Heparin bonding reduces thrombogenicity of pulmonary artery catheters. N Engl J Med 1981; 305: 993–95

19. Lindsay RM, Rourke J, Reid B et al. Platelets, foreign surfaces, and heparin. Trans Am Soc Artif Intern Organs 1976; 22: 292–96

20. Serruys PW, van Hout B, Bonnier H et al. Randomised comparison of implantation of heparin-coated stents with balloon angioplasty in selected patients with coronary artery disease (Benestent II). Lancet 1998; 352: 673–81

21. Vrolix MC, Legrand VM, Reiber JH et al. Heparin-coated Wiktor stents in human coronary arteries (MENTOR trial). MENTOR Trial Investigators. Am J Cardiol 2000; 86: 385–89

22. Wohrle J, Al-Khayer E, Grotzinger U et al. Comparison of the heparin coated vs the uncoated JOSTENT® – no influence on restenosis or clinical outcome. Eur Heart J 2001; 22: 1808–16

23. Sousa JE, Serruys PW, Costa MA. New frontiers in cardiology: drug-eluting stents. Part I. Circulation 2003; 107: 2274–79

24. Klugherz BD, Llanos G, Lieuallen W et al. Twenty-eight-day efficacy and phar-macokinetics of the sirolimus-eluting stent. Coron Artery Dis 2002; 13: 183–88

25. Suzuki T, Kopia G, Hayashi S et al. Stent-based delivery of sirolimus reduces neointimal formation in a porcine coronary model. Circulation 2001; 104: 1188–93

26. Creel CJ, Lovich MA, Edelman ER. Arterial paclitaxel distribution and deposition. Circ Res 2000; 86: 879–84

27. Virmani R, Guagliumi G, Farb A et al. Localized hypersensitivity and late coronary thrombosis secondary to a sirolimus-eluting stent: should we be cautious? Circulation 2004; 109: 701–705

28. Gershlick A, De Scheerder I, Chevalier B et al. Inhibition of restenosis with a paclitaxel-eluting, polymer-free coronary stent: the European evaLUation of pacliTaxel Eluting Stent (ELUTES) trial. Circulation 2004; 109: 487–93

29. Park SJ, Shim WH, Ho DS et al. A paclitaxel-eluting stent for the prevention of coronary restenosis. N Engl J Med 2003; 348: 1537–45

30. Lansky AJ, Costa RA, Mintz GS et al. Non-polymer-based paclitaxel-coated coronary stents for the treatment of patients with de novo coronary lesions: angiographic follow-up of the DELIVER clinical trial. Circulation 2004; 109: 1948–54

31. Kristensen GB, Trope C. Epithelial ovarian carcinoma. Lancet 1997; 349: 113–17

32. Schiff PB, Fant J, Horwitz SB. Promotion of microtubule assembly in vitro by Taxol. Nature 1979; 277: 665–67

33. Rowinsky EK, Donehower RC. Paclitaxel (Taxol). N Engl J Med 1995; 332: 1004–14

34. Nishio K, Arioka H, Ishida T et al. Enhanced interaction between tubulin and microtubule-associated protein 2 via inhibition of MAP kinase and CDC2 kinase by paclitaxel. Int J Cancer 1995; 63: 688–93

35. Rosette C, Karin M. Cytoskeletal control of gene expression: depolymerization of microtubules activates NF-kappa B. J Cell Biol 1995; 128: 1111–19

36. Sollott SJ, Cheng L, Pauly RR et al. Taxol inhibits neointimal smooth muscle cell accumulation after angioplasty in the rat. J Clin Invest 1995; 95: 1869–76

37. Drachman DE, Edelman ER, Seifert P et al. Neointimal thickening after stent delivery of paclitaxel: change in composition and arrest of growth over six months. J Am Coll Cardiol 2000; 36: 2325–32

38. Grube E, Silber S, Hauptmann KE et al. TAXUS I: six- and twelve-month results from a randomized, double-blind trial on a slow-release paclitaxel-eluting stent for de novo coronary lesions. Circulation 2003; 107: 38–42

39. Colombo A, Drzewiecki J, Banning A et al. Randomized study to assess the effectiveness of slow- and moderate-release polymer-based paclitaxel-eluting stents for coronary artery lesions. Circulation 2003; 108: 788–94

40. Heldman AW, Cheng L, Jenkins GM et al. Paclitaxel stent coating inhibits neointimal hyperplasia at 4 weeks in a porcine model of coronary restenosis. Circulation 2001; 103: 2289–95

41. Saunders RN, Metcalfe MS, Nicholson ML. Rapamycin in transplantation: a review of the evidence. Kidney Int 2001; 59: 3–16

42. Gallo R, Padurean A, Jayaraman T et al. Inhibition of intimal thickening after balloon angioplasty in porcine coronary arteries by targeting regulators of the cell cycle. Circulation 1999; 99: 2164–70

43. Poon M, Marx SO, Gallo R et al. Rapamycin inhibits vascular smooth muscle cell migration. J Clin Invest 1996; 98: 2277–83

44. Marx SO, Jayaraman T, Go LO et al. Rapamycin-FKBP inhibits cell cycle regulators of proliferation in vascular smooth muscle cells. Circ Res 1995; 76: 412–17

45. Braun-Dullaeus RC, Mann MJ, Dzau VJ. Cell cycle progression: new therapeutic target for vascular proliferative disease. Circulation 1998; 98: 82–89

46. Marx SO, Marks AR. Bench to bedside: the development of rapamycin and its application to stent restenosis. Circulation 2001; 104: 852–55

47. Gummert JF, Ikonen T, Morris RE. Newer immunosuppressive drugs: a review. J Am Soc Nephrol 1999; 10: 1366–80

48. Schreiber SL. Chemistry and biology of the immunophilins and their immuno-suppressive ligands. Science 1991; 251: 283–87

49. Carter AJ, Falotico R. The sirolimus-eluting Bx VELOCITY™ stent: preclinical data. In Serruys PW, Rensing BJ, eds. Handbook of Coronary Stents. London: Martin Dunitz; 2002: pp. 349–58

50. Farb A, John M, Acampado E et al. Oral everolimus inhibits in-stent neointimal growth. Circulation 2002; 106: 2379–84

51. Virmani R, Jones R, Kar S et al. Everolimus and sirolimus drug-eluting stents are equally effective at reducing neointimal proliferation in a 28-day porcine coronary model, presented at the Transcatheter Cardiovascular Therapeutics 2003. Washington, DC; 2003

52. Grube E, Sonoda S, Ikeno F et al. Six- and twelve-month results from first human experience using everolimus-eluting stents with bioabsorbable polymer. Circulation 2004; 109: 2168–71

53. Costa RA, Grube E, Negoita M et al. Everolimus-eluting stents for the prevention of restenosis: results of the FUTURE II trial. J Am Coll Cardiol 2004; 43: 12A

54. Buellesfeld L, Grube E. ABT-578-eluting stents. The promising successor of sirolimus- and paclitaxel-eluting stent concepts? Herz 2004; 29: 167–70

55. Grube E, Buellesfeld L. Rapamycin analogs for stent-based local drug delivery. Everolimus- and tacrolimus-eluting stents. Herz 2004; 29: 162–66

56. Gerckens U, Silber S, Horstkotte D et al. Evaluation of a tacrolimus-eluting coronary stent graft for treatment of saphenous vein graft lesions: procedural and 6-month follow-up results of the EVIDENT trial, presented at the Transcatheter Cardiovascular Therapeutics 2003. Washington, DC

57. De Scheerder I, Wilczek K, van Dorpe J et al. Local angiopeptin delivery using coated stents reduces neointimal proliferation in overstretched porcine coronary arteries. J Invasive Cardiol 1996; 8: 215–22

58. Armstrong J, Gunn J, Arnold N et al. Angiopeptin-eluting stents: observations in human vessels and pig coronary arteries. J Invasive Cardiol 2002; 14: 230–38

59. Kowk OH, Chow WH, Lee CH et al. First human experience in angiopeptin-eluting stent: preliminary clinical outcome of the Stent With Angiopeptin (SWAN) trial. Am J Cardiol 2002; 90 (Suppl 6A): 72H

60. Kutryk MJ, Foley DP, van den Brand M et al. Local intracoronary administration of antisense oligonucleotide against c-myc for the prevention of in-stent restenosis: results of the randomized investigation by the Thoraxcenter of antisense DNA using local delivery and IVUS after coronary stenting (ITALICS) trial. J Am Coll Cardiol 2002; 39: 281–87

61. Kipshidze NN, Iversen P, Kim HS et al. Advanced c-myc antisense (AVI-4126)-eluting phosphorylcholine-coated stent implantation is associated with complete vascular healing and reduced neointimal formation in the porcine coronary restenosis model. Catheter Cardiovasc Interv 2004; 61: 518–27

62. Liu X, Huang Y, Hanet C et al. Study of antirestenosis with the BiodivYsio® dexamethasone-eluting stent (STRIDE): a first-in-human multicenter pilot trial. Catheter Cardiovasc Interv 2003; 60: 172–78

63. Geraldes P, Sirois MG, Bernatchez PN et al. Estrogen regulation of endothelial and smooth muscle cell migration and proliferation: role of p38 and p42/44 mitogen-activated protein kinase. Arterioscler Thromb Vasc Biol 2002; 22: 1585–90

64. New G, Moses JW, Roubin GS et al. Estrogen-eluting, phosphorylcholine-coated stent implantation is associated with reduced neointimal formation but no delay in vascular repair in a porcine coronary model. Catheter Cardiovasc Interv 2002; 57: 266–71

65. Abizaid A, Albertal M, Costa MA et al. First human experience with the 17-beta-estradiol-eluting stent: the Estrogen And Stents To Eliminate Restenosis (EASTER) trial. J Am Coll Cardiol 2004; 43: 1118–21

66. De Smet BJ, de Kleijn D, Hanemaaijer R et al. Metalloproteinase inhibition reduces constrictive arterial remodeling after balloon angioplasty: a study in the atherosclerotic Yucatan micropig. Circulation 2000; 101: 2962–67

67. Gobeil F, Laflamme M, Bouchard M et al. BiodivYsio® stent coated with metallo-proteinase inhibitor reduces neointimal hyperplasia in a porcine coronary artery restenosis model. Circulation 2001; 104: II–388

68. Aggarwal RK, Ireland DC, Azrin MA, Ezekowitz MD, de Bono DP, Gershlick AH. Antithrombotic potential of polymer-coated stents eluting platelet glycoprotein IIb/IIIa receptor antibody. Circulation 1996; 94: 3311–317

69. Alt E, Haehnel I, Beilharz C et al. Inhibition of neointima formation after experimental coronary artery stenting: a new biodegradable stent coating releasing hirudin and the prostacyclin analog iloprost. Circulation 2000; 101: 1453–458

# PART II

# TREATMENT OF RESTENOSIS

# 4. Trials of Oral Drug Therapy to Reduce Restenosis

Jose A Silva

## Introduction

The development of drug-eluting stents (DES) has dramatically reduced the incidence of restenosis after percutaneous coronary intervention (PCI). Randomized trials have demonstrated that the sirolimus- and paclitaxel-eluting coronary stents decrease the 6-month restenosis rate to less than 10%.[1–3] Nevertheless, DES have yet to be tested in more complex lesions. It is possible that unfavorable lesion characteristics, such as the presence of calcification, fibrosis, organized thrombus, etc, may decrease the diffusion or penetration of the drug into the vessel layers rendering the DES less effective in this complex milieu. Under these circumstances the use of a systemic approach to deliver antiproliferative drug may be an attractive therapeutic option.

Multiple systemic pharmacologic approaches have been tested in attempting to decrease the restenosis rate after stent placement with negative results.[4] Probucol, a lipid-lowering agent, was the first medication to show promising results in reducing restenosis after stand-alone balloon angioplasty.[5,6] In addition, recent studies, have demonstrated that the use of two oral medications – rapamycin and cilostazol – do inhibit intimal proliferation and decreases the restenosis rate after balloon angioplasty and stent placement.[7,8] In this chapter we will address the most important pharmacologic actions of these three drugs and present the results of some clinical trials that have shown the positive effect of these medications in restenosis rate.

## Mechanisms of action

### Probucol

Prior to its withdrawal from the market in the USA, probucol had been used for the treatment of hypercholesterolemia for several decades. Although its mechanism of action was not completely clear, the drug proved to be very effective in reducing LDL cholesterol and, unlike other lipid-lowering agents, probucol did not require functioning LDL receptors to lower LDL cholesterol, rendering it effective for the treatment of familial hypercholesterolemia.[9,10] Probucol is also a potent antioxidant, which limits vascular oxidative stress and superoxide generation.[11] It is believed that these antioxidant properties selectively inhibit LDL degradation in macrophage-rich fatty streaks and slow progression of atherosclerosis, which is independent of its anti-atherogenic effects related to reduction of LDL cholesterol.[12] Despite its LDL cholesterol-lowering activity, probucol was never considered a first-line medication because it also lowers the HDL cholesterol by 20 to 30%, in addition to having side-effects in the gastrointestinal system and prolonging the Q-T interval in the electrocardiogram.[9]

## Rapamycin

Rapamycin (sirolimus; Rapamune®) is a macrocyclic lactone produced by *Streptomyces hygroscopicus*. It inhibits T-lymphocyte activation and proliferation that occurs in response to antigenic and cytokine stimulation, particularly interleukine (IL)-2, IL-4, and IL-5 by a mechanism that differs from other immunosuppressants. Rapamycin binds FK binding protein-12 (FKBP-12) and the complex inhibits the activation of a key regulatory kinase, the mammalian Target Of Rapamycin (mTOR). This inhibition in turn suppresses cytokine-driven T-cell proliferation and its progression from the $G_1$ to the S phase of the cell cycle. This profound inhibition of proliferation, migration, and inflammation make this agent useful in treating acute renal allograft rejection and allograft arteriopathy (Table 4.1).[13] Animal studies have shown that the systemic administration of rapamycin is highly effective in decreasing intimal proliferation and restenosis after balloon angioplasty.[14]

## Cilostazol

Cilostazol (Pletal®) is a quinolone derivative that inhibits cellular phosphodiesterases, particularly phosphodiesterase III. This inhibition leads to suppression of cAMP degradation, leading to an increased level of cAMP in platelets and blood vessels, and resulting in platelet inhibition and vasodilation. Cilostazol reversibly inhibits platelet aggregation induced by thrombin, ADP, collagen, arachidonic acid, epinephrine, and shear stress.[15] Cilostazol also inhibits smooth muscle proliferation and neointimal formation after balloon injury in vascular models.[16] This drug has also been shown to produce non-homogeneous dilation of different vascular beads, preferentially the femoral arteries, with less – although still significant – effect in the carotid, vertebral, and mesenteric arteries, and negligible effect in the renal arteries. In the heart cilostazol has been shown to increase the heart rate, and increase myocardial contractility in animal models. It also causes a reduction of triglycerides, and an increase in HDL (see Table 4.1).[15]

# Clinical studies

## Probucol

Probucol was shown to decrease restenosis after balloon angioplasty in several small clinical studies.[5,6] In one prospective randomized trial, 317

**Table 4.1. Oral drug therapy for restenosis**

|  | Rapamycin | Cilostazol |
| --- | --- | --- |
| Name | Sirolimus; Rapamune® | Pletal® |
| Chemical structure | Macrocyclic lactone derived from Streptomyces hygroscopicus | Quinolone |
| Mechanism of action | ↓ T lymphocytes activation and proliferation<br>↓ Antibody production<br>↓ Activation of mTOR and cytokine-driven T-cell proliferation in the progression from the $G_1$ to the S phase of cell cycle | Inhibits cellular phosphodiesterases<br>Inhibits cAMP in platelets (↓ aggregation) and blood vessels (vasodilation)<br>↓ Smooth muscle proliferation<br>↓ Neointimal formation after balloon injury<br>↓ Triglycerides; ↑ HDL |
| Clinical indications | Acute renal allograft rejection and allograft arteriopathy | Intermittent claudication |
| Metabolism | Substrate of cytochrome P-450 and P-glycoprotein<br>Excreted in the feces (91%) and kidney (2–3%) | Substrate of cytochrome P-450 (active metabolites)<br>Active metabolites excreted in the urine |
| Dose | Loading dose: 6 mg orally<br>Maintenance dose: 2 to 5 mg orally | 50 to 150 mg orally<br>100 mg orally b.i.d.<br>Dose adjustment: with ketoconazole, erythromycin, diltiazem, omeprazole |
| Adverse reactions | Incidence: 3–20% per year<br>Asthenia; constipation; diarrhea; edema<br>↑ Cholesterol and triglycerides levels<br>Renal and hepatic dysfunction<br>Leucopenia; thrombocytopenia | Incidence: 25–30% usually transient; nausea, diarrhea, headaches, palpitations, dizziness |

patients were assigned to four groups: 1, placebo; 2, probucol; 3, multivitamins; or 4, probucol and multivitamins.[6] The binary restenosis rates and late loss were significantly lower in the two groups that received probucol (Figure 4.1). Of note, treatment with probucol and/or multivitamins was started four weeks prior to balloon angioplasty, which appears to be important to obtain the benefit, since the study that started with probucol immediately prior to intervention did not find a restenosis benefit.[17] The same investigators later reported, in an intravascular ultrasound study, that the decrease in restenosis rate conferred by this medication was mainly exerted by improving vascular remodeling with this medication.[18]

Although in-vitro and animal studies have shown that probucol has important antiproliferative effects in smooth muscle cells after balloon injury

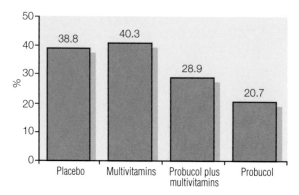

**Figure 4.1:** Restenosis rates in patients receiving placebo, probucol, multivitamins, or combination, showing significantly lower restenosis rates in the two groups receiving probucol (P = 0.003 probucol versus no probucol).

by promoting endothelialization[19] or by induction of heme oxygenase-1,[20] clinical studies have not shown this lipid-lowering agent to decrease neointimal thickening or the restenosis rate after coronary stent placement.[21,22]

## Rapamycin

Three recent coronary trials using oral rapamycin have demonstrated that this medication decreases intimal proliferation and in-stent restenosis in de-novo lesions.[23–25] In one study,[23] oral rapamycin was given to 30 patients with type A or B1 de-novo lesions (3–4 mm in diameter, <25 mm in length) with stable or unstable angina. All patients received a 6-mg oral loading dose, followed by 2 mg daily for 2 weeks (15 patients) or 4 weeks (15 patients). The late loss was 0.48 ± 0.44 mm and the restenosis rate was 9.1%.

In the Oral Rapamune to Inhibit Restenosis (ORBIT) study,[24] 60 patients with non-complex coronary lesions were reported. All patients received an oral loading dose of 5 mg, followed by 2 mg (30 patients) or 5 mg daily (30 patients) for 30 days. Three patients in the 2-mg group, and 9 patients in the 5-mg group discontinued the drug due to skin rash, diarrhea, mouth ulcers, or fatigue, or a combination of these symptoms. At the six-month angiographic follow-up, there was no difference in late loss (0.62 ± 0.61 mm vs 0.68 ± 0.56 mm, P = 0.56) or binary restenosis (7.1% vs 6.9%; P = 0.97) between the 2-mg and the 5-mg groups. This luminal late loss is superior to historical controls (0.8–1.1 mm) but inferior to the luminal late loss obtained with DES (0.1–0.2 mm) (Figure 4.2). In the Oral Rapamycin in Argentina (ORAR) study,[25] 76 patients and 103 arteries were treated with an oral loading dose of 6 mg followed by a maintenance dose of 2 mg daily for 4 weeks. Patients who attained a serum rapamycin level >8 ng/ml had significantly lower late loss (0.65 mm vs 1.11 mm; P = 0.03) and a lower binary restenosis rate (6.2% vs 23%; P = 0.04), compared to those patients with a serum rapamycin level ≤8 ng/ml.

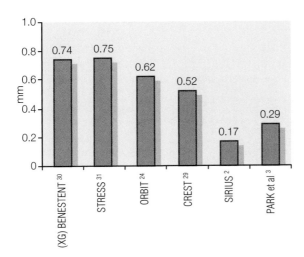

Figure 4.2: Late coronary luminal loss in six-stent trial of bare metal stents,[30,31] oral rapamycin and cilostazol,[24,29] and DES.[2,3]

In contrast to the favorable results observed in these three preliminary studies, a recent report found no benefit when oral rapamycin was used for the treatment of 22 coronary patients with recalcitrant in-stent restenosis.[26] These patients had been treated an average of 3.5 times with PCI for this condition prior to enrollment, and 20 of 22 patients had already failed brachytherapy. In addition, 11 patients (50%) needed to discontinue the medication due to side-effects including leukopenia ($n = 3$), hyper-triglyceridemia ($n = 3$), abnormal liver function tests ($n = 1$), and minor symptoms ($n = 4$). This experience is different from the three studies mentioned previously in that no side-effects or discontinuation of the drug were reported in the first study ($n = 30$), and only three of 100 patients needed to discontinue the drug in the second study.[24,25]

## Cilostazol

Cilostazol (Pletal®; Otsuca, America Pharma, Inc, Rockville, MD) is a type III phosphodiesterase inhibitor, approved by the FDA for the treatment of peripheral arterial disease and intermittent claudication. Several prospective placebo-controlled trials have shown that cilostazol improves the walking distance in patients with mild-to-moderate intermittent claudication.[27] The proposed mechanisms leading to clinical benefit in claudication of this drug are vasodilation, smooth muscle relaxation, enhanced effect of prostacyclin, and inhibition of platelet activity.[15]

Cilostazol has also been shown to have strong antiproliferative properties, leading to a decrease in the restenosis rate after balloon angioplasty or stents in animal models.[16] The beneficial effect on restenosis after balloon angioplasty has been demonstrated in the coronary circulation. In a study of 211 patients randomized to cilostazol or placebo after balloon angioplasty, the group that received cilostazol developed less restenosis (using

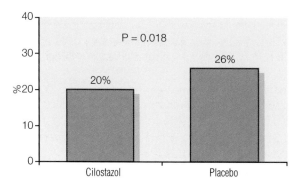

Figure 4.3: Restenosis rates in the CREST trial comparing cilostazol to placebo. The Cilostazol for Restenosis (CREST) investigators recently presented their results of 705 patients randomized to coronary stent placement with cilostazol for six months or placebo.[29]

quantitative coronary angiography) and less target vessel revascularization, compared to the group that received placebo.[28] The Cilostazol for Restenosis (CREST) investigators recently presented their results of 705 patients randomized to coronary stent placement with cilostazol for six months or placebo (Figure 4.3).[29] The group that received cilostazol had a late loss of 0.52 mm compared with 0.70 mm in the placebo group (P = 0.018). The binary restenosis rate was 20.9% for the cilostazol-treated patients, compared to 34.6% for placebo group (P = 0.0006). Subgroup analysis of diabetic patients revealed less restenosis in the cilostazol-treated group (17%), compared with placebo (37%; P = 0.01).

## Conclusion

Multiple drugs have been tested systemically in an attempt to reduce the restenosis rate after balloon angioplasty and coronary stent placement. So far, only three oral medications (probucol, rapamycin, and cilostazol) have been shown to reduce restenosis after PCI. Probucol, begun at least four weeks prior to intervention, appears to reduce restenosis after balloon angioplasty by favorably affecting vascular remodeling after percutaneous transluminal coronary angioplasty; however, no effect has been shown following stent placement. In contrast, oral rapamycin and cilostazol have been shown to decrease intimal proliferation compared to placebo. These drugs appear reasonably safe and well tolerated by most patients. In the case of oral rapamycin and cilostazol, the magnitude of the reduction in intimal hyperplasia appears to be 'intermediate' to that of DES. It remains to be seen whether these drugs will prove useful in clinical practice, or whether they might further decrease the restenosis rate when used in conjunction with DES.

# References

1. Morice AC, Serruys PW, Sousa JE et al. A randomized comparison of a sirolimus-eluting stent with a standard stent for coronary revascularization. N Engl J Med 2002; 346: 1773–80

2. Moses JF, Leon MB, Popma JJ et al. Sirolimus-eluting stents versus standard stents in patients with stenosis in a native coronary artery. N Engl J Med 2003; 349: 1315–23

3. Park SJ, Shim WH, Ho DS et al. A paclitaxel-eluting stent for the prevention of coronary restenosis. N Engl J Med 2003; 348: 1537–45

4. Faxon DP. Systemic drug therapy for restenosis. "Déjà vu all over again". Circulation 2002; 106: 2296–98

5. Watanabe K, Sekiya M, Ikeda S et al. Preventive effects of probucol on restenosis after percutaneous transluminal coronary angioplasty. Am Heart J 1996; 132: 23–29

6. Tardiff JC, Cote G, Lesperance J et al. Probucol and multivitamins in the prevention of restenosis after coronary angioplasty. N Engl J Med 1997; 337: 365–72

7. Gallo R, Padurean A, Jayaraman T et al. Inhibition of intimal thickening after balloon angioplasty in porcine coronary arteries by targeting regulators of the cell cicle. Circulation 1999; 99: 2164–70

8. Kubota Y, Kichikawa K, Uchida H et al. Pharmacologic treatment of intimal hyperplasia after metallic stent placement in the peripheral arteries. An experimental study. Invest Radiol 1995; 30(9): 532–37

9. Nestruck AC, Bouthillier D, Sing CF et al. Apoliprotein E polymorphism and plasma cholesterol response to probucol. Metabolism 1987; 36(8): 743–47

10. Kita T, Nagano Y, Yokode M et al. Probucol prevents the progression of atherosclerosis in the Watanabe heritable hyperlipidemic (WHHL) rabbit, an animal model for familial hypercholesterolemia. Proc Natl Acad Sci USA 1987; 84: 5928–31

11. Keaney JF Jr, Xu A, Cunningham D et al. Dietary probucol preserves endothelial function in cholesterol-fed rabbits by limiting vascular oxidative stress and superoxide generation. J Clin Invest 1995; 95: 2520–29

12. Carew TE, Schwenke DC, Steinberg D. Anti-atherogenic effect of probucol unrelated to its hypocholesterolemic effect: evidence that antioxidants in vivo can selectively inhibit low-density lipoprotein degradation in macrophage-rich fatty streaks and slow the progression of atherosclerosis in the Watanabe heritable hyperlipidemic rabbit. Proc Natl Acad Sci USA 1987; 84: 7725–29

13. Saunders RN, Metcalfe MS, Nicholson ML. Rapamycin in transplantation: a review of evidence. Kidney Int 2001; 59: 3–16

14. Gallo R, Padurean A, Jayaraman T et al. Inhibition of intimal thickening after balloon angioplasty in porcine coronary arteries by targeting regulators of the cell cycle. Circulation 1999; 99: 2164–70

15. Sorkin EM, Markham A. Cilostazol: new drug profile. Drugs Aging 1999; 14: 63–71

16. Matzumoto Y, Tani T, Watanabe K et al. Effects of cilostazol, an antiplatelet drug, on smooth muscle cell proliferation after endothelial denudation in rats. Jpn J Pharmacol 1992 (Suppl 1): 284P

17. O'Keefe JH, Stone GW, McCallister BD Jr et al. Lovastatin plus probucol for prevention of restenosis after percutaneous transluminal coronary angioplasty. Am J Cardiol 1996; 77: 649–52

18. Cote G, Tardiff JC, Lesperance J et al. Effects of probucol on vascular remodeling after coronary angioplasty. Circulation 1999; 99: 30–35

19. Lau AK, Leichtweis SB, Hume P et al. Probucol promotes functional re-endothelialization in balloon-injured rabbit aortas. Circulation 2003; 107: 2031–36

20. Deng YM, Wu BJ, Witting PK et al. Probucol protects against smooth muscle cell proliferation by upregulating heme oxygenase-1. Circulation 2004; 110: 1855–60

21. Tardiff JC, Gregoire J, Schwartz L et al. Effects of AGI-1067 and probucol after percutaneous coronary interventions. Circulation 2003; 107: 552–58

22. Kim MH, Cha KS, Han JY et al. Effect of antioxidant probucol for preventing stent restenosis. Cathet Cardiovasc Intervent 2002; 57: 424–28

23. Mehran R, Marx S, Kesanacurthy S et al. Oral rapamycin for the prevention of in-stent restenosis. J Am Coll Cardiol 2003; 41: 74A

24. Waksman R, Ajani A, Pichard AD et al. Oral rapamycin to inhibit restenosis after stenting of de-novo coronary lesions. The Oral Rapamune to Inhibit Restenosis (ORBIT) study. J Am Coll Cardiol 2004; 44: 1386–92

25. Rodriguez AE, Rodriguez-Alemparte M, Fernandez-Pereira C et al. Oral rapamycin in patients undergoing coronary stent therapy: final results of the ORAR study (Oral Rapamycin in Argentina). J Am Coll Cardiol 2004; 43: 102A

26. Brara PS, Moussavian M, Grise MA et al. Pilot trial of oral rapamycin for recalcitrant restenosis. Circulation 2003; 107: 1722–24

27. Dawson DL, Cutler BS, Meissner MH et al. Cilostazol has beneficial effects in treatment of intermittent claudication: results from a multicenter, randomized prospective, double-blind trial. Circulation 1998; 98: 678–86

28. Tsuchikane E, Fukuhara A, Kobayashi T et al. Impact of cilostazol on restenosis after percutaneous coronary balloon angioplasty. Circulation 1999; 100: 1058–66

29. Douglas JS, Holmes DR, Kereiakes D et al. Cilostazol for restenosis (CREST) trial. A randomized, double-blind study following coronary artery stent implantation. Circulation 2003; 108: 4

30. Serruys PW, de Jaegere P, Kiemeneij F et al. A comparison of balloon-expandable stent implantation with balloon angioplasty in patients with coronary artery disease. N Engl J Med 1994; 331: 489–95

31. Fishman D, Leon MB, Baim D et al. A randomized comparison of coronary stent placement and balloon angioplasty in the treatment of coronary disease. N Engl J Med 1994; 331: 496–501

# 5. NON-STENT DEVICES TO REDUCE RESTENOSIS

## Srinivasa P Potluri and Jose A Silva

### Introduction

Percutaneous transluminal coronary angioplasty (PTCA) has been an accepted alternative to surgical revascularization in selected cases, since its introduction by Andres Gruntzig 25 years ago.[1] The major limitation of this technique is restenosis; the use of endovascular stents have definitely improved the late patency for percutaneous procedures but recurrent stenosis remains a significant limitation.

In this chapter the most pertinent clinical studies of the non-stent mechanical approaches to decrease restenosis will be reviewed. This includes devices for debulking lesions, and brachytherapy, which has been the only non-stent technology proved to be highly effective to decrease restenosis.

### Directional coronary atherectomy

Directional coronary atherectomy (DCA) was approved by the US Food and Drug Administration (FDA) for coronary use in 1990 as the first non-balloon percutaneous coronary intervention (PCI) device (Figure 5.1). Directional coronary atherectomy was designed to remove atheroma with directional control. Studies with DCA and intravascular ultrasound (IVUS) suggested that tissue removal accounts for 50 to 70% of the luminal enlargement after DCA.

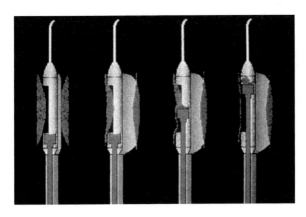

**Figure 5.1:** Directional coronary atherectomy catheter.

## Clinical trials of directional coronary atherectomy

The Coronary Atherectomy Versus Angioplasty Trial (CAVEAT-I) was the first randomized trial comparing DCA with PTCA in de-novo lesions of native coronary arteries (Table 5.1).[2] The six-month restenosis rate was not significantly lower in the DCA group (50% vs 57%; P = 0.06), but the complication rate (composite of any myocardial infarction, death, or CABG 11% vs 5%; P < 0.05) was significantly higher in the DCA group. The Canadian Coronary Atherectomy Trial (CCAT) compared DCA with PTCA in proximal left anterior descendent (LAD) lesions in 274 patients and showed no significant reduction in angiographic (43% vs 46%) or clinical restenosis (30.1% vs 30.6%).[3] A similar lack of benefit in the restenosis rate was demonstrated in the Coronary Atherectomy versus Angioplasty Trial (CAVEAT-II) in saphenous vein graft lesions (see Table 5.1).[4] In this trial the DCA group also had a higher incidence of major adverse cardiac events (MACE) compared to the PTCA group (20.1% for DCA and 12.2% for PTCA; P < 0.05).

After the negative results of these trials, proponents of the technique questioned whether the lack of benefit of DCA over PTCA to decrease the restenosis rate was due to an insufficient plaque-removal technique, and they hypothesized that a more aggressive plaque-removal approach would improve the results.[5] In the Optimal Atherectomy Restenosis Study (OARS), 199 patients underwent 'optimal' DCA to achieve less than 15% residual

| Table 5.1. Randomized trials of directional coronary atherectomy | | | | |
|---|---|---|---|---|
| Trial | Comparison | Patients (n) | Restenosis | Clinical outcome (MACE) |
| CAVEAT-I[2] | DCA vs PTCA | 1012 | 50% vs 57%; P = 0.06 | 8.6% vs 4.6%; P = 0.007 |
| CCAT[3] | DCA vs PTCA in LAD | 274 | 46% vs 43%; P = 0.7 | Non-significant |
| CAVEAT-II[4] | DCA vs PTCA in SVG | 305 | 46% vs 51%; P = 0.41 | TLR trended to be low in PTRA; P = 0.09 |
| BOAT[40] | Optimal DCA vs PTCA | 989 | 31% vs 40%; P = 0.02 | Non-significant |
| START[9] | DCA vs stenting | 122 | 16% vs 33%; P = 0.03 | 19% vs 34%; P = 0.06 |
| AMIGO[11] | DCA + stent vs stent alone | 753 | 27% vs 22%; P = 0.2 | Non-significant |

DCA, directional coronary atherectomy; LAD, left anterior descending coronary artery; PTCA, percutaneous transluminal coronary angioplasty; SVG, saphenous vein graft; TLR, target lesion revascularization.

diameter stenosis.[6,7] Using this aggressive plaque debulking technique resulted in a six-month restenosis rate of 28.9%, substantially lower than for the CAVEAT trial.

The improved success and safety of DCA in the OARS study led to the Balloon vs Optimal Atherectomy Trial (BOAT) which enrolled 1000 patients with a single de-novo coronary lesion and randomized patients to either optimal DCA (residual stenosis <20%) or PTCA.[8] The primary end-point was the six-month angiographic restenosis rate at 6, which was significantly lower for the DCA group (31.4% vs 39.8%; P = 0.016). However, target vessel revascularization (TVR) was not different between the groups (25% vs 28%; P = non-significant, NS). The BOAT trial also showed that the one-year mortality rate was not different in the DCA group compared to the PTCA group (0.6% vs 1.6%; P = NS). Overall, this trial demonstrated a modest decrease in angiographic restenosis but no clinical advantage for patients treated with DCA compared to PTCA.

A smaller study – the STent versus directional coronary Atherectomy Randomized Trial (START) – compared bare metal stent (BMS) placement to optimal DCA and found that restenosis at 6 months (32.8% vs 15.8%; P = 0.032), and target vessel failure (33.9% vs 18.3%; P = 0.056) at one year were lower in the DCA group.[9] This study has not been confirmed in larger multicenter randomized trials.

The concept of plaque debulking with DCA prior to stent placement was tested in the Stenting after Optimal Lesion Debulking (SOLD) study, which suggested that this strategy might have a positive impact on late patency with a restenosis rate of 11% and target lesion revascularization (TLR) of 7% at a mean follow-up of 18 months.[10] The AMIGO trial compared a strategy of DCA debulking prior to stent placement to stent placement alone in a prospective randomized trial of 753 patients. No differences were found for angiographic restenosis (26.7% for DCA plus stenting, versus 22.1% for stenting alone; P = 0.237) or in clinical outcomes.[11]

In conclusion, the marginal benefit of a debulking strategy with DCA is highly dependent on operator experience. The data do not support the use of DCA alone or DCA debulking prior to stent placement over standard techniques such as stand-alone PTCA or stent placement.

## Percutaneous transluminal rotational atherectomy

Percutaneous transluminal rotational atherectomy (PTRA) was developed as a second-generation device to specifically address calcified lesions known to be difficult to treat with PTCA alone (Figure 5.2). The technique utilizes a high-speed rotating elliptical burr coated with a fine diamond abrasive to achieve plaque ablation of the relatively hard and inelastic components of the atherosclerotic plaque. Since its introduction in 1990, the rotational atherectomy device has undergone several design modifications and changes in the procedural technique.

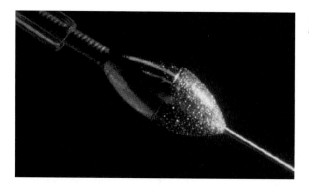

Figure 5.2: Rotational atherectomy: Rotablator®.

## Clinical trials

### PTRA versus PTCA

The Excimer laser, Rotational atherectomy, and Balloon Angioplasty Comparison (ERBAC) study was the first randomized trial to compare PTRA with PTCA.[12] A total of 685 patients with complex coronary lesions were randomly assigned to balloon angioplasty ($n = 222$), excimer laser angioplasty ($n = 232$), or rotational atherectomy ($n = 231$). The primary end-point was procedural success (diameter stenosis <50%, absence of death, Q-wave myocardial infarction, and coronary artery bypass surgery). The procedural success rate of the PTRA group was higher than the laser angioplasty and balloon angioplasty (89% vs 77% and 80%; P = 0.002) groups; however, the six-month TVR was higher in the PTRA group (42.4%) than in the laser (46.0%) or balloon angioplasty groups (31.9%; P = 0.013).

In another study – the Comparison Of Balloon versus Rotational Angioplasty (COBRA) trial – 502 patients with complex coronary lesions were prospectively randomized to PTCA or PTRA.[13] The procedural success (80% vs 76%; P = NS) and the six-month restenosis rate (37% vs 35%; P = NS) were comparable in the PTRA and the PTCA groups, respectively. In addition, the Dilatation versus Ablation Revascularization Trial Targeting Restenosis (DART) study, comparing PTRA with PTCA in 446 patients failed to show any benefit for rotational atherectomy compared to balloon angioplasty in procedural success, angiographic restenosis, or TVR (Table 5.2).[14] The data from these trials suggest that PTRA may yield a marginally higher procedural success rate than stand-alone balloon angioplasty when treating complex calcified lesions; however, the use of PTRA does not decrease restenosis rates or TVR.

### PTRA versus adjunctive stenting

The use of stents following PTRA or PTCA was evaluated in the Stenting POst Rotational atherectomy Trial (SPORT) study.[15] This study randomized 735 patients with calcified lesions to PTRA with stenting versus PTCA with

**Table 5.2. Randomized trials of percutaneous rotational atherectomy (Rotablator®)**

| Trial | Comparison | Patients (n) | Restenosis | Clinical outcome (MACE) |
|---|---|---|---|---|
| ERBAC[12] | PTRA vs PTCA | 453 | 57% vs 47%; P = 0.1 | 46% vs 37%; P = 0.04 |
| COBRA[13] | PTRA vs PTCA | 502 | 49% vs 51%; P = 0.3 | Non-significant |
| DART[14] | PTRA vs PTCA in small vessels | 446 | 51% vs 51%; P = 0.1 | Non-significant |
| SPORT[15] | PTRA with stent vs stenting | 735 | 18% vs 15%; P = NS | Non-significant |
| ROSTER[17] | PTRA vs PTCA in ISR | 200 | 32% vs 45%; P = 0.04 | Non-significant |
| ARTIST[18] | PTRA vs PTCA in ISR | 298 | 65% vs 51%; P = 0.04 | 20% vs 9%; P = 0.005 |

ISR, in-stent restenosis; PTCA, percutaneous transluminal coronary angioplasty; PTRA, percutaneous transluminal rotational angioplasty.

stenting. Although the post-procedure luminal gain was higher in PTRA and stenting group, the acute complications were the same and the TVR at 6 months was no better with PTRA (18% vs 15%; P = NS).

## PTRA for treatment of in-stent restenosis

Rotational atherectomy has also been employed for the treatment of in-stent restenosis. Two studies suggested that lesion debulking with PTRA decreased the restenosis rate compared to PTCA alone. In a non-randomized multicenter registry of 304 patients, the Balloon Angioplasty or Rotational Atherectomy in the treatment of intra-STEnt Restenosis (BARASTER) study compared tissue debulking with PTRA followed by PTCA, to PTCA alone, or PTRA alone and found reduced rates of one-year clinical events (death, myocardial infarction, and TLR) (PTRA and PTCA 38% vs PTCA alone 52% vs PTRA alone 60%).[16]

These results led to a randomized trial – the ROtational atherectomy versus balloon angioplasty for diffuse in-STEnt Restenosis (ROSTER) study – which included 200 patients with in-stent restenosis (ISR) >10 mm long.[17] The 12-month TLR was significantly lower in the PTRA group compared to the PTCA group (32% vs 45%; P = 0.04). However, the decrease in TLR of rotational atherectomy compared with balloon angioplasty alone found in the ROSTER study, was not confirmed in a larger prospective randomized trial: the Angioplasty versus Rotational atherectomy of the Treatment of diffuse In-Stent restenosis Trial (ARTIST).[18] In this study, 298 patients with lesions

10–50 mm across were randomized to PTRA with PTCA, or PTCA alone. The six-month angiographic restenosis rate (65% vs 51%; P = 0.04) and TLR (48% vs 36%; P = 0.06) were higher for the PTRA group.

In conclusion, two prospective randomized trials comparing PTRA versus PTCA for the treatment of in-stent restenosis have yielded opposite results. Based on these data, a strategy of PTRA ± PTCA over balloon angioplasty alone for the treatment of ISR does not appear justified (see Table 5.2).

## Cutting balloon angioplasty

The cutting balloon (CB) is a non-compliant balloon with metal cutting blades mounted on its surface (Figure 5.3). The CB theoretically reduces vessel stretch and vessel injury by scoring the vessel longitudinally rather than causing random disruption of the atherosclerotic plaque. This mechanism of 'controlled injury' with the metal blades not only allows the treatment of resistant (undilatable) lesions but some investigators also believed that it might decrease the restenosis rate compared to an 'uncontrolled injury' created by the standard balloon angioplasty.

### Clinical trials

In the Cutting balloon Angioplasty versus Plain old balloon Angioplasty randomized Study (CAPAS) 232 patients were randomized to cutting balloon angioplasty (CBA) or PTCA in type B or C lesions and small arteries.[19] The restenosis rate was significantly lower (25.2% vs 41.5%; P = 0.009) in the CBA group. At one-year follow-up, the event-free survival was 72.8% in the CBA group and 61.0% in the PTCA group (P = 0.047). This study suggested that CBA provided superior angiographic and clinical outcomes compared to PTCA in small coronary arteries.

However, the benefits of CBA over plain old balloon angioplasty (POBA) was not confirmed in the Global Randomized Trial, the largest multicenter randomized clinical trial that compared CBA with PTCA for the treatment of

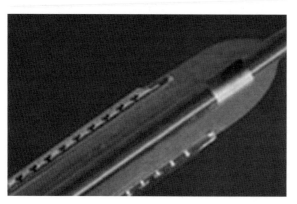

Figure 5.3: Cutting balloon: a balloon with microblades which score the plaque and relax it as it is compacted by the balloon.

**Table 5.3. Randomized trials of cutting balloon angioplasty**

| Trial | Comparison | Patients (n) | Restenosis | Clinical outcome (MACE) |
|-------|-----------|--------------|------------|-------------------------|
| CAPAS[19] | CBA vs PTCA | 232 | 25% vs 42%; P = 0.009 | 27% vs 39%; P = 0.047 |
| GRT[20] | CBA vs PTCA | 1238 | 31% vs 30%; P = 0.75 | 14% vs 15%; P = 0.34 |
| RESCUT[22] | CBA vs PTCA for ISR | 428 | 30% vs 31%; P = 0.82 | Non-significant |

CBA, cutting balloon angioplasty; ISR, in-stent restenosis; PTCA, percutaneous transluminal coronary angioplasty.

de-novo type A or B lesions in a native coronary artery.[20] A total of 1238 patients (1385 lesions) were randomized to CBA or PTCA. The angiographic restenosis rate at six months (31% vs 30.4%; P = NS) and MACE at nine months of follow-up (10% vs 12.9%; P = NS) were not different between CBA and POBA (Table 5.3).

Cutting balloon angioplasty has been suggested as a treatment for ISR.[21] The only randomized trial to assess ISR (RESCUT) compared the CBA with PTCA in 428 patients with ISR.[22] At seven months of follow-up, the restenosis rate was not different between the groups (CBA 29.8%, PTCA 31.4%; P = 0.82), with a similar pattern of recurrent restenosis. The clinical event rates at seven months of follow-up were also similar in both groups.

A post-hoc analysis of the Radiation in Europe with Novoste (RENO) registry of ISR treated with CBA or PTCA prior to coronary beta radiation recently showed that the CBA patients had a lower six-month TLR (10.2% vs 16.6%, respectively; P = 0.04; and MACE odds ratio 0.49; P = 0.02).[23] These favorable results of CBA prior to brachytherapy have yet to be confirmed in a randomized trial.

In conclusion, CBA does not reduce the restenosis rate or MACE when treating ISR, compared with conventional PTCA. No randomized controlled study supports the use of CB to reduce recurrent stenosis for de-novo or restenotic lesions (see Table 5.3).

## Laser-assisted coronary angioplasty

Laser-assisted coronary angioplasty, with a paucity of efficacy data, has been approved for the treatment of saphenous vein graft (SVG) lesions, chronic total occlusions, calcified, ostial, and long lesions (>20 mm), as well as PTCA failures. Despite these indications, widespread use of laser-assisted coronary angioplasty has been limited, due to a significant incidence of dissections and perforations, and negative results from randomized trials (Table 5.4).

| Table 5.4. Randomized trials of laser angioplasty | | | | |
|---|---|---|---|---|
| Trial | Comparison | Patients (n) | Restenosis | Clinical outcome (MACE) |
| AMRO[24] | LA vs PTCA | 308 | 52% vs 41%; P = 0.1 | Non-significant |
| ERBAC[12] | LA vs PTCA | 454 | 46% vs 32%; P = 0.01 | Not analyzed |
| LAVA[25] | LA vs PTCA | 215 | Not reported | Non-significant |

LA, laser angioplasty; PTCA, percutaneous transluminal coronary angioplasty.

## Clinical trials

In the Amsterdam–Rotterdam trial (AMRO), 308 patients with lesions longer than 10 mm were randomized to laser or PTCA.[24] Major cardiovascular events at six months of follow-up were 33% for laser and 30% for balloon angioplasty. In the ERBAC trial, 620 patients with type B and C coronary lesions were randomized to laser, PTCA, or PTRA.[12] The procedural success was 88%, 84%, and 93%, respectively. The incidence of major complications was greater with the excimer laser than with rotational atherectomy or balloon angioplasty. At the six-month follow-up, revascularization of the original target lesion was performed more frequently in the rotational atherectomy group (42.4%) and the excimer laser group (46.0%) than in the angioplasty group (31.9%; P = 0.013).

In the Laser Angioplasty Versus Angioplasty (LAVA) trial, using a mid-infrared holmium:yttrium–aluminum–garnet (YAG) laser, 215 patients were randomized to laser or PTCA.[25] The procedural success rates were similar in both groups; however, the rate of major and minor procedural complications (18.0% vs 3.1%; P = 0.0004), myocardial infarctions (4.3% vs 0%; P = 0.04), and total in-hospital major adverse events (10.3% vs 4.1%; P = 0.08) was significantly higher in the laser angioplasty group. At a mean follow-up of 11.2 ± 7.7 months, there were no differences in event-free survival in patients assigned to laser treatment or PTCA. Laser-assisted angioplasty has also been used to treat ISR. However, late patency rates have varied widely among reports and no randomized trials are available (see Table 5.4).

In conclusion, compared to stand-alone PTCA, laser-assisted PTCA results in a more complicated hospital course without short-term or long-term benefits. There is no evidence that the use of the laser lowers restenosis rates after PCI.

## Coronary brachytherapy

Vascular brachytherapy following PTCA for the prevention of restenosis was introduced in 1992, and in November 2000 the FDA approved its use for the treatment of ISR. Vascular brachytherapy is delivered as gamma or beta radiation. Several trials have proven the effectiveness of vascular brachytherapy to decrease restenosis following PTCA. Indeed, this has been the only effective treatment modality for restenosis prior to the development of DES. Below we will briefly discuss the most important results of these clinical trials.

## Clinical trials of gamma radiation

The first report of human experience with gamma radiation came from Venezuela where 21 patients were treated with intracoronary radiation with [192]Ir to assess its safety and feasibility. The restenosis rate was 28.6% at six months of follow-up and remained unchanged after five years. The angiographic complications included the formation of four coronary aneurysms which did not further enlarge or rupture after three years of follow-up.

The Study of Coronary Radiation to Inhibit Proliferation Post-Stenting (SCRIPPS) was the first randomized trial that evaluated the safety and efficacy of intracoronary gamma radiation given as adjunctive therapy to stent placement (Figure 5.4).[26] In this study, 26 of 55 patients received [192]Ir at a prescribed dose of 8–30 Gy with a dwell time of 20–45 minutes. The stenosis rate at 6.8 months of follow-up was significantly lower in the radiation group (17% vs 54%; P = 0.01). The three-year follow-up available in 67% of the patients revealed 33% restenosis in radiation group versus 64% in placebo group (P < 0.05). Following the SCRIPPS trial, the SCRIPPS II for ISR in diffuse lesions, SCRIPPS III with prolonged antiplatelet therapy (clopidogrel for 6–12 months), and SCRIPPS IV trials to evaluate high-dose radiation were initiated (Table 5.5).

In the Washington Radiation for In-Stent restenosis Trial (WRIST) 130 patients (100 native ISR and 30 with SVG ISR) were randomized to [192]Ir or

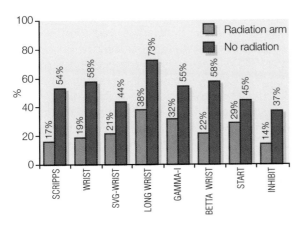

Figure 5.4: Six-month restenosis rate. The binary restenosis rates for the radiation arm were significantly (P<0.05) lower in all trials. However, the MACE and survival results did not achieve statistical significance.

| Table 5.5. Randomized trials of gamma brachytherapy for ISR | | | | | |
|---|---|---|---|---|---|
| Trial | Comparison | Patients (n) | Primary end-point (experimental standard) | Restenosis (experimental vs standard) | Summary |
| SCRIPPS[26] | Radiation vs placebo for ISR | 55 | Binary stenosis | 17% vs 54%; P = 0.01 | MACE was 15% vs 48%; P = 0.01 at 1 year |
| WRIST[27] | Radiation vs placebo for ISR | 130 | Binary stenosis at 6 months | 19% vs 58%; P = 0.0001 | Significant reduction in MACE and TLR |
| SVG-WRIST[28] | Radiation vs placebo for ISR in SVG | 120 | MACE at 12 months | 21% vs 44%; P = 0.005 at 6 months | MACE and TLR were significantly lower at 12 months |
| LONG WRIST[29] | Radiation vs placebo for long ISR (36–80 mm) | 120 | MACE at 12 months | 38% vs 73%; P < 0.05 at 6 months | MACE was lower with 15 Gy and further lower with 18 Gy (P < 0.05) |
| GAMMA-I[31] | Radiation vs placebo for ISR (dose ranging) | 252 | MACE at 9 months | 32% vs 55% | MACE was lower, although it was driven by decreased TLR with higher MIs in treated patients due to late thrombosis |

Gy, Gray; ISR, in-stent restenosis; MACE, major adverse coronary events; MI, myocardial infarction; SVG, saphenous vein graft; TLR, target lesion revascularization.

placebo.[27] The six-month angiographic restenosis rate was significantly lower in the irradiated group (19% vs 58%; P = 0.0001). Likewise, MACE and the TLR rates were significantly lower in the irradiated group. To test the effectiveness of brachytherapy in reducing the ISR rate in SVG, the SVG-WRIST study randomized 120 patients with vein graft ISR to brachytherapy or placebo.[28] The restenosis rate, as well as MACE and TLR at six months were also significantly lower in the brachytherapy group compared to placebo (21% vs 44%; P = 0.02; 32% vs 63%; P < 0.001; and 17% vs 57%; P = 0.001, respectively).

The LONG WRIST for long lesions randomized 120 patients with diffuse ISR 36–80 mm long to brachytherapy or placebo.[29] The six-month restenosis rate (32% vs 71%; P = 0.0002), MACE (38% vs 62%; P = 0.01), and TLR (30% vs 60%; P = 0.001) rates were all significantly lower in the brachytherapy group. The WRIST PLUS study was designed to answer the question of whether a prolonged regimen (six months) of clopidogrel plus aspirin would decrease the risk of late-stent thrombosis.[30] The results of this study showed that longer antiplatelet therapy reduces late stent thrombosis from 9.6% to 2.5% (P = 0.02). The WRIST-12 was initiated to examine the benefit of 12 months of clopidogrel. The group treated with 12 months of antiplatelet therapy had a rate of 21% for MACE and 20% for target-lesion revascularization compared with 36% (P = 0.01) and 35% (P = 0.009), respectively, in patients who were treated with only six months of clopidogrel.[30]

Similarly, GAMMA-I was a multicenter randomized trial evaluating the [192]Ir gamma-radiation dosimetry using IVUS (8–30 Gy).[31] They randomized 252 patients and found at six months that there was significantly lower restenosis with greatest benefit in patients with long lesions and diabetes. After nine months, MACE was significantly lower in the irradiated group (28% vs 44%; P = 0.02). The rate of death and acute MI were not significantly higher in the irradiated group (3.12 vs 0.8; P = 0.17; and 9.9% vs 4.1%; P = 0.09, respectively). The results of these trials have conclusively demonstrated the efficacy of intracoronary gamma radiation with [192]Ir for the treatment and prevention of ISR.

## Clinical trials of beta radiation for ISR

The BETA WRIST registry examined the efficacy of beta radiation for ISR in 50 patients.[27] The clinical outcomes were compared between these patients and those of the original placebo arm of the WRIST cohort; the restenosis rate was 22%. When compared to the restenosis rate of the placebo arm of the original WRIST trial, the treated patients in the BETA WRIST registry demonstrated a 58% reduction in TLR at six months (P < 0.001).

A pivotal multicenter, randomized trial – the STents And Radiation Therapy (START) – involved 476 patients and was designed to determine the efficacy and safety of the Beta Cath system (Novoste Corporation, Norcross, GA).[32] At eight months of follow-up the restenosis rates were 24% for the irradiated and 46% for the placebo group (P < 0.001). In the irradiated group, TLR was 13% compared to 22% in controls (P = 0.008) (Table 5.6).

### Table 5.6. Clinical trials of beta brachytherapy for ISR

| Trial | Comparison | Patients (n) | Primary end-point (experimental standard) | Restenosis (experimental vs standard) | Summary |
|---|---|---|---|---|---|
| BETA WRIST[27] | Radiation vs control arm of original WRIST | 50 | Binary restenosis | 22% vs 58%; P = 0.001 | Reduction in MACE and TLR similar to original WRIST |
| START[32] | Radiation vs placebo | 476 | TVR at 8 months | 29% vs 45%; P = 0.001 | 8 month MACE and TVR were significantly lower |
| INHIBIT[34] | Radiation vs placebo | 332 | MACE and binary stenosis at 9 months | 14% vs 37%; P = 0.0001 | MACE and TVR were significantly lower in radiation group |

MACE, major adverse coronary events; TVR, target vessel revascularization.

The START 40/20 trial was a 207-patient registry designed to ensure an adequate irradiation margin, with an additional 10 mm of radiation therapy covering the proximal and the distal edges of the interventional injury.[33] When compared to the control arm of the START trial, the START 40/20 showed a 44% reduction in restenosis (P = 0.002), a 34% reduction in TLR (P = 0.03), and a 26% reduction in MACE (P = 0.001). The START 40/20 registry showed no deleterious effects of adding an additional 10 mm of radiation to the edges. The INtimal Hyperplasia Inhibition with Beta Instent Trial (INHIBIT) examined the efficacy of the Galileo (Guidant Corporation, Indianapolis, IN) radiation therapy system in 332 patients and the primary safety end-point of death, MI, or repeat target-lesion revascularisation over 290 days (15% vs 31%; P = 0.0006).[34] The angiographic restenosis rate was lower in the radiated group than the placebo group for the entire lesion segment (14% vs 31%; P < 0.0001).

The Beta Radiation to prevent In-sTEnt restenosis (BRITE) trial was a feasibility study to test the RDX (Radiance Medical Systems, Irvine, CA) coronary radiation system (which uses a balloon catheter encapsulating a sleeve of $^{32}$P for treatment of ISR) which showed the lowest reported binary stenosis rates (7.7%) in 27 patients.[35] To confirm these results BRITE II, a randomized multicenter trial, has been initiated.

In conclusion, clinical trials have demonstrated the efficacy of intracoronary beta radiation brachytherapy for decreasing restenosis rates. However, there was no relationship between the reduced restenosis rates and clinical outcomes, probably due to the 'geographic miss' phenomenon, edge effects ('candy-wrapper effect'), and late thrombosis (see Figure 5.4).

## Clinical trials of beta radiation for de-novo lesions

Clinical studies investigating the effectiveness of beta radiation for de-novo, restenotic, and ISR lesions have been similar to the encouraging results of gamma radiation. The Geneva trial confirmed the safety and feasibility of beta radiation for de-novo lesions.[36] The Beta Energy Restenosis Trial (BERT) was a dose-testing trial.[37] The Beta Radiation In Europe (BRIE) registry of 149 patients showed a TVR rate of 22% and 31% at six months and one year of follow-up, respectively.[38] In BRIE, inadequate coverage of the injured segment by the radioactive source or geographical miss affected 67.9% of the vessels, which led to an increase in edge restenosis, compared to the group in whom geographical miss did not occur (16.3% vs 4.3%; P = 0.004). Geographic miss was responsible for 40% of the treatment failures.

The BETA CATH trial was the first prospective randomized trial using the $^{90}$Sr/Y source train, and showed a similar eight-month TLR and MACE between the radiation and placebo groups. This study was also the first to identify a higher-than-expected rate of late stent thrombosis when radiation was used with additional stent implantation. The Proliferation REduction with Vascular ENergy Trial (PREVENT) randomized 105 patients with de-novo

**Table 5.7. Randomized trials of brachytherapy in de-novo coronary lesions**

| Trial | Comparison | Patients (n) | Primary end-point (experimental standard) | Restenosis (experimental vs standard) | Summary |
|---|---|---|---|---|---|
| BETA CATH[27] | Radiation + PTCA or stent vs PTCA or stent alone | 1100 | 8 month TLR | 15% vs 14%; P = 0.4 | Sub-analysis showed significant decrease in TLR in PTCA group |
| PREVENT[39] | Radiation + PCI vs PCI alone | 80 of 105 | 12 month MACE | 8% vs 39%; P = 0.01 at the target site | MACE was not significantly different at 12 months |

MACE, major adverse coronary event; PCI, percutaneous coronary intervention; PTCA, percutaneous transluminal coronary angioplasty; TLR, target lesion revascularization.

(70%) or restenotic (30%) lesions to placebo or different doses of beta radiation with $^{32}$P.[39] The binary restenosis rate at six months was 8.2%, and 39% (P = 0.001) at the target site, and 22.4% and 50% (P = 0.02) for the segment (target site plus the adjacent segment) in the treated and the placebo groups, respectively. Major cardiovascular events were not different (16% vs 24%; P = NS). It also showed a paradoxically positive treatment effect in the lesion segment and a negative treatment effect in the analysis segment which may have been due to geographic miss (Table 5.7).

In summary, brachytherapy for de-novo coronary lesions is safe and feasible although it has not been shown to decrease late clinical end-points. Two radiotherapy-related problems were identified: arterial stenosis adjacent to the edge of the target site; and late coronary thrombo-occlusive events. The use of longer radiotherapy sources which provide a wide margin of treatment beyond the segment of injury may overcome the problem of geographic miss and edge narrowing. Prolonged use of antiplatelet agents and avoiding the use of new stents should minimize the occurrence of late thrombotic events.

## References

1. Gruntzig A. Transluminal dilatation of coronary-artery stenosis. Lancet 1978; 1(8058): 263
2. Topol EJ, Leya F, Pinkerton CA et al. A comparison of directional atherectomy with coronary angioplasty in patients with coronary artery disease. The CAVEAT Study Group. N Engl J Med 1993; 329(4): 221–27
3. Adelman AG, Cohen EA, Kimball BP et al. A comparison of directional atherectomy with balloon angioplasty for lesions of the left anterior descending coronary artery. N Engl J Med 1993; 329(4): 228–33

4. Holmes DR Jr, Topol EJ, Califf RM et al. A multicenter, randomized trial of coronary angioplasty versus directional atherectomy for patients with saphenous vein bypass graft lesions. CAVEAT-II Investigators. Circulation 1995; 91(7): 1966–74

5. Baim DS, Kuntz RE. Directional coronary atherectomy: how much lumen enlargement is optimal? Am J Cardiol 1993; 72(13): 65E–70E

6. Simonton CA, Leon MB, Baim DS et al. 'Optimal' directional coronary atherectomy: final results of the Optimal Atherectomy Restenosis Study (OARS). Circulation 1998; 97(4): 332–39

7. Simonton CA. Directional coronary atherectomy: optimal atherectomy trials and new combined strategies with coronary stents. Semin Interv Cardiol 2000; 5(4): 193–98

8. Baim DS, Hinohara T, Holmes D et al. Results of directional coronary atherectomy during multicenter preapproval testing. The US Directional Coronary Atherectomy Investigator Group. Am J Cardiol 1993; 72(13): 6E–11E

9. Tsuchikane E, Sumitsuji S, Awata N et al. Final results of the STent versus directional coronary Atherectomy Randomized Trial (START). J Am Coll Cardiol 1999; 34(4): 1050–57

10. Moussa I, Moses J, Di Mario C et al. Stenting after optimal lesion debulking (SOLD) registry. Angiographic and clinical outcome. Circulation 1998; 98(16): 1604–609

11. Stankovic G, Colombo A, Bersin R et al. Comparison of directional coronary atherectomy and stenting versus stenting alone for the treatment of de novo and restenotic coronary artery narrowing. Am J Cardiol 2004; 93(8): 953–58

12. Reifart N, Vandormael M, Krajcar M et al. Randomized comparison of angioplasty of complex coronary lesions at a single center. Excimer Laser, Rotational Atherectomy, and Balloon Angioplasty Comparison (ERBAC) study. Circulation 1997; 96(1): 91–98

13. Dill T, Dietz U, Hamm CW et al. A randomized comparison of balloon angioplasty versus rotational atherectomy in complex coronary lesions (COBRA study). Eur Heart J 2000; 21(21): 1759–66

14. Mauri L, Reisman M, Buchbinder M et al. Comparison of rotational atherectomy with conventional balloon angioplasty in the prevention of restenosis of small coronary arteries: results of the Dilatation vs Ablation Revascularization Trial Targeting Restenosis (DART). Am Heart J 2003; 145(5): 847–54

15. Bittl JA, Chew DP, Topol EJ et al. Meta-analysis of randomized trials of percutaneous transluminal coronary angioplasty versus atherectomy, cutting balloon atherotomy, or laser angioplasty. J Am Coll Cardiol 2004; 43(6): 936–42

16. Goldberg SL, Berger P, Cohen DJ et al. Rotational atherectomy or balloon angioplasty in the treatment of intra-stent restenosis: BARASTER multicenter registry. Catheter Cardiovasc Interv 2000; 51(4): 407–13

17. Sharma SK, Kini A, Mehran R et al. Randomized trial of Rotational Atherectomy Versus Balloon Angioplasty for Diffuse In-stent Restenosis (ROSTER). Am Heart J 2004; 147(1): 16–22

18. Vom Dahl J, Dietz U, Haager PK et al. Rotational atherectomy does not reduce recurrent in-stent restenosis: results of the angioplasty versus rotational

atherectomy for treatment of diffuse in-stent restenosis trial (ARTIST). Circulation 2002; 105(5): 583–88

19. Izumi M, Tsuchikane E, Funamoto M et al. Final results of the CAPAS trial. Am Heart J 2001; 142(5): 782–89

20. Mauri L, Bonan R, Weiner BH et al. Cutting balloon angioplasty for the prevention of restenosis: results of the Cutting Balloon Global Randomized Trial. Am J Cardiol 2002; 90(10): 1079–83

21. Albiero R, Nishida T, Karvouni E et al. Cutting balloon angioplasty for the treatment of in-stent restenosis. Catheter Cardiovasc Interv 2000; 50(4): 452–59

22. Albiero R, Silber S, Di Mario C et al. Cutting balloon versus conventional balloon angioplasty for the treatment of in-stent restenosis: results of the restenosis cutting balloon evaluation trial (RESCUT). J Am Coll Cardiol 2004; 43(6): 943–49

23. Roguelov C, Eeckhout E, De Benedetti E, et al. Clinical outcome following combination of cutting balloon angioplasty and coronary beta-radiation for in-stent restenosis: a report from the RENO registry. J Invasive Cardiol 2003; 15(12): 706–9.

24. Appelman YE, Koolen JJ, Piek JJ et al. Excimer laser angioplasty versus balloon angioplasty in functional and total coronary occlusions. Am J Cardiol 1996; 78(7): 757–62

25. Stone GW, de Marchena E, Dageforde D et al. Prospective, randomized, multicenter comparison of laser-facilitated balloon angioplasty versus stand-alone balloon angioplasty in patients with obstructive coronary artery disease. The Laser Angioplasty Versus Angioplasty (LAVA) Trial Investigators. J Am Coll Cardiol 1997; 30(7): 1714–21

26. Teirstein PS, Massullo V, Jani S et al. Catheter-based radiotherapy to inhibit restenosis after coronary stenting. N Engl J Med 1997; 336(24): 1697–703

27. Waksman R, Bhargava B, White L et al. Intracoronary beta-radiation therapy inhibits recurrence of in-stent restenosis. Circulation 2000; 101(16): 1895–98

28. Waksman R, Ajani AE, White RL et al. Intravascular gamma radiation for in-stent restenosis in saphenous-vein bypass grafts. N Engl J Med 2002; 346(16): 1194–99

29. Waksman R, Cheneau E, Ajani AE et al. Intracoronary radiation therapy improves the clinical and angiographic outcomes of diffuse in-stent restenotic lesions: results of the Washington Radiation for In-Stent Restenosis Trial for Long Lesions (Long WRIST) Studies. Circulation 2003; 107(13): 1744–49

30. Waksman R, Ajani AE, Pinnow E et al. Twelve versus six months of clopidogrel to reduce major cardiac events in patients undergoing gamma-radiation therapy for in-stent restenosis: Washington Radiation for In-Stent restenosis Trial (WRIST) 12 versus WRIST PLUS. Circulation 2002; 106(7): 776–78

31. Leon MB, Teirstein PS, Moses JW et al. Localized intracoronary gamma-radiation therapy to inhibit the recurrence of restenosis after stenting. N Engl J Med 2001; 344(4): 250–56

32. Popma JJ, Suntharalingam M, Lansky AJ et al. Randomized trial of 90Sr/90Y beta-radiation versus placebo control for treatment of in-stent restenosis. Circulation 2002; 106(9): 1090–96

33. Suntharalingam M, Laskey W, Lansky AJ et al. Clinical and angiographic outcomes after use of 90Strontium/90Yttrium beta radiation for the treatment of in-stent restenosis: results from the Stents and Radiation Therapy 40 (START 40) registry. Int J Radiat Oncol Biol Phys 2002; 52(4): 1075–82

34. Waksman R, Raizner AE, Yeung AC et al. Use of localised intracoronary beta radiation in treatment of in-stent restenosis: the INHIBIT randomised controlled trial. Lancet 2002; 359(9306): 551–57

35. Waksman R, Buchbinder M, Reisman M et al. Balloon-based radiation therapy for treatment of in-stent restenosis in human coronary arteries: results from the BRITE I study. Catheter Cardiovasc Interv 2002; 57(3): 286–94

36. Verin V, Popowski Y, de Bruyne B et al. Endoluminal beta-radiation therapy for the prevention of coronary restenosis after balloon angioplasty. The Dose-Finding Study Group. N Engl J Med 2001; 344(4): 243–49

37. King SB 3rd, Williams DO, Chougule P et al. Endovascular beta-radiation to reduce restenosis after coronary balloon angioplasty: results of the beta energy restenosis trial (BERT). Circulation 1998; 97(20): 2025–30

38. Serruys PW, Sianos G, van der Giessen W et al. Intracoronary beta-radiation to reduce restenosis after balloon angioplasty and stenting; the Beta Radiation In Europe (BRIE) study. Eur Heart J 2002; 23(17): 1351–59

39. Raizner AE, Oesterle SN, Waksman R et al. Inhibition of restenosis with beta-emitting radiotherapy: Report of the Proliferation Reduction with Vascular Energy Trial (PREVENT). Circulation 2000; 102(9): 951–58

40. Baim DS, Cutlip DE, Sharma SK et al. Final results of the Balloon vs Optimal Atherectomy Trial (BOAT). Circulation 1998; 97(4): 322–31

# 6. Clinical Trials of Bare Metal Stents to Reduce Restenosis

## Jose A Silva

## Introduction

Coronary stent placement has revolutionized the field of interventional cardiology over the past decade. It has taken almost 20 years from the first implantation of a coronary stent in a human for this technique to become safe, effective, and widely accepted. At present, coronary stents are implanted in the majority of all percutaneous coronary interventions (PCI).

The initial obstacle that investigators had to overcome with these devices was the problem of stent thrombosis. Initial series showed that stent thrombosis occurred in up to 20% of all cases, leading to unacceptably high myocardial infarction (MI) and mortality rates.[1] Due to this high peri-procedural stent thrombosis rate, patients were treated with aggressive anticoagulation regimens, which in turn led to frequent bleeding complications. For this reason, stents were only used as a bail-out procedure, for the treatment of abrupt occlusion after balloon angioplasty.[2] In 1995, Colombo and colleagues demonstrated that optimal stent expansion using a technique of high pressure balloon inflation, dramatically reduced the incidence of stent thrombosis to less than 2%.[3] This technique also replaced coumadin with antiplatelet agents, ticlopidine, and aspirin, which led to a dramatic reduction in bleeding complications.

The results of two trials showing that the restenosis rate after coronary stent placement was significantly lower than after balloon angioplasty alone,[4,5] followed by Colombo's landmark study,[3] marked the beginning of the 'stent era'. After the results of these studies were published, the use of coronary stents grew exponentially, and the indications expanded steadily over the next few years. Last year, approximately 900 000 coronary stents were placed worldwide, and it is believed that their use will continue to grow as the population continues to age and as technology continues to improve, particularly with the development of drug-eluting stents (DES).

In this chapter we will address the impact of coronary stents in decreasing restenosis in native coronary arteries and bypass graft de-novo lesions, restenosis lesions, abrupt occlusions, chronic occlusions, and acute MI, situations in which there is clear consensus for using these devices.

## Elective stent placement of focal de-novo native coronary lesions

Coronary stents were proven to decrease the restenosis rate compared to balloon angioplasty alone in two prospective randomized trials of native coronary arteries (Figure 6.1).[4,5] In the STent REStenosis Study (STRESS), 410 patients with symptomatic coronary disease and reference vessels over 3.0 mm in diameter and less than 15 mm in length were randomized to elective stent placement or balloon angioplasty.[4] The six-month binary restenosis rate was 31.6% for the stent group and 42.1% for the balloon angioplasty group (P = 0.046). Target vessel revascularization (TVR) and major adverse cardiovascular events (MACE) were 10.2% and 15.4% for the stent and balloon angioplasty groups, respectively (P = 0.06).

In the BElgium NEtherlands STENT (BENESTENT I) trial, 520 patients were randomized to elective stenting or balloon angioplasty (see Figure 6.1).[5] The patients treated with coronary stent placement had a significantly lower restenosis rate at six months of follow-up compared to patients treated with balloon angioplasty (22% vs 32%; P = 0.02). In these two trials the bleeding complications were slightly, although non-statistically, higher in the stent group, compared to balloon angioplasty, probably due to the fact that aggressive anticoagulation was still routinely used in the stent group. In the BENESTENT II trial, 827 patients with coronary ischemia were randomized to revascularization with heparin-coated stents or balloon angioplasty alone.[6] At six-month follow-up, the restenosis rate was significantly lower in the stent group (16% vs 31%; P = 0.0008) and the composite of death, MI, and TVR was 12.8% in the stent group, compared to 19.3% in the balloon angioplasty group (P = 0.013). In this study ticlopidine and aspirin were used instead of warfarin, and the bleeding complications were low (1.2% and 1.0%) in both groups.

With these three landmark studies, the efficacy of stent placement to reduce the restenosis rates was conclusively demonstrated. In addition, it was shown that stent revascularization was safe and carried no more bleeding complications or abrupt occlusion than balloon angioplasty alone.

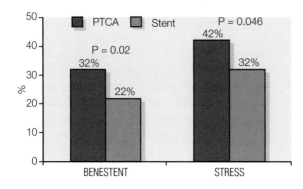

Figure 6.1: Bare metal stent compared to balloon angioplasty for six-month restenosis.

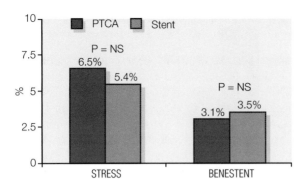

Figure 6.2: Thirty-day death and myocardial infarction rates comparing bare metal stents and balloon angioplasty. NS, non-significant.

Interestingly, these studies did not demonstrate that stent placement was safer than balloon angioplasty when the 30-day death and MI rates were compared (Figure 6.2).

## Abrupt or threatened occlusion

Balloon angioplasty leads to tearing of the vessel wall, luminal enlargement, and fragmentation of the atherosclerotic plaque. This trauma inflicted in the vessel wall, may cause dissection of the intima and/or media, which, when combined with the elastic recoil that follows balloon dilation, may culminate in abrupt or threatened arterial occlusion. After balloon angioplasty, abupt or threatened occlusion occurs in approximately 5% of the patients, and carries a significant morbidity and mortality.[2] Before the advent of endovascular stents, the treatment of this condition included prolonged balloon inflation, often with a perfusion balloon catheter, or emergency coronary bypass surgery. By scaffolding the vessel wall and sealing the dissection, stents proved more effective than prolonged balloon inflation as a bail-out treatment for abrupt or threatened occlusion.

Furthermore, stent placement was shown not only to be highly effective in restoring immediate patency of the occluded vessel, but also proved to decrease the restenosis rate compared to balloon angioplasty in randomized trials (Figure 6.3). In the Trial of Angioplasty and Stents in Canada (TASC II), patients were randomized to prolonged balloon inflation or stenting after abrupt vessel occlusion.[7] Even though about 25% of the balloon angioplasty patients crossed over to bail-out stenting, the six-month restenosis rate was 50% for the prolonged balloon inflation group and 22% for the bail-out stenting group (P = 0.02). Similar benefits of stent placement were demonstrated in the STENT-BY study in which 100 patients were randomized to prolonged balloon inflation or bail-out stenting. In this study, the six-month restenosis rate in the balloon inflation group was 65% and for the bail-out stenting group 24% (P = 0.01).[8]

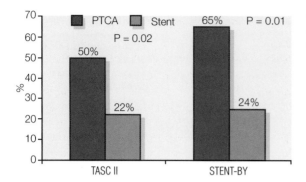

Figure 6.3: Restenosis rates for balloon angioplasty versus bail-out stenting.

## Saphenous vein grafts

Conventional balloon angioplasty of atherosclerotic vein graft lesions is limited by the risk of distal embolization of plaque during intervention and by a high restenosis rate of 50 to 70%.[9] Except for stent placement in these conduits, other technologies such as directional atherectomy (DCA) or atherectomy with the transluminal extraction catheter (TEC) have been disappointing.[10,11]

Non-randomized studies and retrospective data have suggested that stent placement in saphenous vein grafts (SVGs) lowers the restenosis rate and decreases MACE in these patients. In the SAVED trial (Stent versus balloon Angioplasty for aortocoronary saphenous VEin bypass graft Disease) – the only prospective randomized study comparing Palmaz–Schatz stenting with balloon angioplasty in focal SVG lesions – the freedom from MACE was higher in the stent group (73% vs 58%; P = 0.03) but there was no significant difference in the binary restenosis rates (Figure 6.4).[12] Coronary stent placement is therefore indicated for all SVG lesions felt to be amenable to a catheter-based approach.

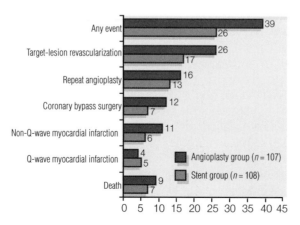

Figure 6.4: The SAVED trial: major cardiac events up to 240 days post-procedure.[12]

## Restenotic lesions after balloon angioplasty

Stand-alone balloon angioplasty is performed relatively infrequently at present, due to its high restenosis rate. However, when restenotic lesions are treated with a second balloon dilation, the likelihood for restenosis is higher than when treating de-novo lesions. Stent placement has been shown to decrease the restenosis rate compared to stand-alone balloon angioplasty in these circumstances. In the Restenosis Stent Study (REST), 383 patients with restenotic lesions were randomized to revascularization with balloon angioplasty or Palmaz–Schatz stents.[13] The group treated with stents had a significantly lower restenosis rate than the group treated with balloon angioplasty (32% vs 18%; P = 0.002).

## Chronic total occlusion

The restenosis rate after percutaneous revascularization with stand-alone balloon angioplasty of chronic total occlusion is approximately 50%. Several prospective randomized trials have shown that the restenosis rate and clinical events rate can be substantially decreased with stent revascularization compared to balloon angioplasty alone (Figure 6.5).[14–18] Based on these data, stent placement is considered the percutaneous treatment of choice for chronic total occlusions.

## Acute myocardial infarction

Mechanical reperfusion, when available, is the preferred treatment to restore normal coronary flow and to decrease cardiac mortality in patients with acute ST elevation MI (STEMI).[19] Despite the advantages of percutaneous intervention over intravenous thrombolysis, primary angioplasty is limited by a reocclusion rate of 10 to 15% and a restenosis rate of 30 to 50%.[20] Although acute MI was initially considered a contraindication to stent placement due to a theoretical increased likelihood for stent thrombosis, high-pressure balloon inflation, and the routine use of antiplatelet agents (a thienopyridine in

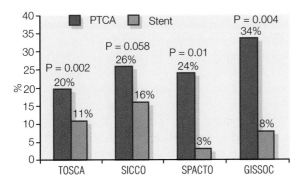

Figure 6.5: (a) Reocclusion rate after revascularization of chronic total occlusion;

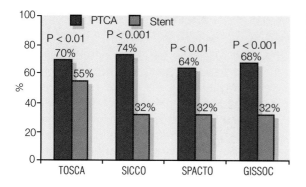

(b) restenosis rate after revascularization of chronic total occlusions;

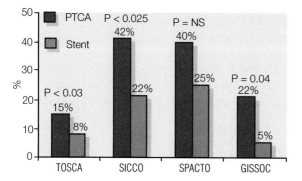

(c) TVR rate after revascularization of chronic total occlusions. NS, non-significant.

combination with aspirin), or more recently of platelet IIb/IIIa inhibitors, has proved that stents can be safely implanted in a thrombotic milieu.

Several prospective randomized trials have demonstrated that stent placement decreases the in-hospital and long-term MACE and restenosis rate compared to primary balloon angioplasty for the treatment of STEMI. In the PAMI stent trial 900 patients with acute STEMI were randomized to mechanical reperfusion with primary balloon angioplasty ($n = 448$) or primary stenting ($n = 452$).[21] At six months of follow-up the restenosis rate and TVR were significantly lower in the primary stenting group (Figure 6.6). In the Comparison of Angioplasty with Stenting, with or without abciximab, in Acute Myocardial Infarction (CADILLAC) Trial, 2082 patients with acute STEMI presenting within 12 hours of symptom onset were randomized to primary angioplasty or primary stent placement with and without abciximab.[22] At six months of follow-up, the primary end-point, a composite of death, reinfarction, disabling stroke, and ischemia-driven revascularization occurred in 20% after PTCA, 16.5% after PTCA plus abciximab, 11.5% after stenting, and 10.2% after stenting plus abciximab (P < 0.001). The difference in the incidence of

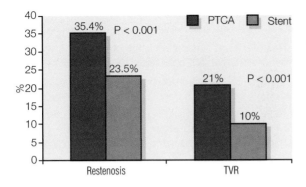

Figure 6.6: PAMI stent trial (*n* = 900) at six-month follow-up.[21]

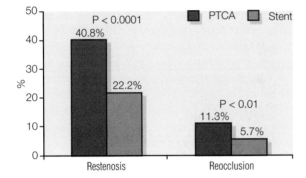

Figure 6.7: Six-month restenosis and reocclusion rates of the CADILLAC trial.[22]

primary end-point was due entirely to differences in the rates of TVR. The six-month binary restenosis rates were also significantly lower in the primary stent group (Figure 6.7). These prospective randomized trials have proved that when feasible, primary stent placement is the treatment of choice for STEMI.

## Conclusion

Percutaneous coronary intervention with stent implantation has emerged as the preferred percutaneous revascularization modality in interventional cardiology. Many prospective randomized trials have shown that stent revascularization yields superior procedural success, lower MACE rates, and lower restenosis rates than balloon angioplasty alone in the treatment of de-novo and restenotic lesions in native coronary arteries, SVGs, abrupt occlusions, chronic total occlusions, and acute MI. It is very likely that with the development of DES the indications for the use of coronary stents will continue to expand and challenge other treatment modalities, particularly surgical revascularization.

# References

1. Serruys PW, Strauss BH, Beatt KJ et al. Angiographic follow-up after placement of a self-expanding coronary-artery stent. N Engl J Med 1991; 324(1): 13–17

2. Roubin GS, Cannon AD, Agrawal SK et al. Intracoronary stenting for acute and threatened closure complicating percutaneous transluminal coronary angioplasty. Circulation 1992; 85(3): 916–27

3. Colombo A, Hall P, Nakamura S et al. Intracoronary stenting without anticoagulation accomplished with intravascular ultrasound guidance. Circulation 1995; 91(6): 1676–88

4. Fischman DL, Leon MB, Baim DS et al. A randomized comparison of coronary-stent placement and balloon angioplasty in the treatment of coronary artery disease. Stent Restenosis Study Investigators. N Engl J Med 1994; 331(8): 496–501

5. Serruys PW, de Jaegere P, Kiemeneij F et al. A comparison of balloon-expandable stent implantation with balloon angioplasty in patients with coronary artery disease. Benestent Study Group. N Engl J Med 1994; 331(8): 489–95

6. Serruys PW, van Hout B, Bonnier H et al. Randomised comparison of implantation of heparin-coated stents with balloon angioplasty in selected patients with coronary artery disease (Benestent II). Lancet 1998; 352(9129): 673–81

7. Ricci D, Ray S, Buller CE et al. Six-month follow-up of patients randomized to prolonged inflation or stent for abrupt occlusion during PTCA: Clinical and angiographic data – TASC II. Circulation 1995; 92(Suppl 1): 475A

8. Haude M, Erbel R, Hopp H et al. A prospective randomized trial comparing immediate stenting versus conservative treatment strategies in abrupt vessel closure or symptomatic dissections during coronary balloon angioplasty. Eur Heart J 1996; 17 (Suppl): 172A

9. De Feyter PJ, van Suylen RJ, de Jaegere PP et al. Balloon angioplasty for the treatment of lesions in saphenous vein bypass grafts. J Am Coll Cardiol 1993; 21(7): 1539–49

10. Holmes DR Jr., Topol EJ, Califf RM et al. A multicenter, randomized trial of coronary angioplasty versus directional atherectomy for patients with saphenous vein bypass graft lesions. CAVEAT-II Investigators. Circulation 1995; 91(7): 1966–74

11. Twidale N, Barth CW 3rd, Kipperman RM et al. Acute results and long-term outcome of transluminal extraction catheter atherectomy for saphenous vein graft stenoses. Catheter Cardiovasc Diagn 1994; 31(3): 187–91

12. Savage MP, Douglas JS Jr, Fischman DL et al. Stent placement compared with balloon angioplasty for obstructed coronary bypass grafts. Saphenous Vein De Novo Trial Investigators. N Engl J Med 1997; 337(11): 740–47

13. Erbel R, Haude M, Hopp HW et al. Coronary-artery stenting compared with balloon angioplasty for restenosis after initial balloon angioplasty. Restenosis Stent Study Group. N Engl J Med 1998; 339(23): 1672–78

14. Buller CE, Dzavik V, Carere RG et al. Primary stenting versus balloon angioplasty in occluded coronary arteries: the Total Occlusion Study of Canada (TOSCA). Circulation 1999; 100(3): 236–42

15. Sirnes PA, Golf S, Myreng Y et al. Sustained benefit of stenting chronic coronary occlusion: long-term clinical follow-up of the Stenting in Chronic Coronary Occlusion (SICCO) study. J Am Coll Cardiol 1998; 32(2): 305–10

16. Hoher M, Wohrle J, Grebe OC et al. A randomized trial of elective stenting after balloon recanalization of chronic total occlusions. J Am Coll Cardiol 1999; 34(3): 722–29

17. Rubartelli P, Verna E, Niccoli L et al. Coronary stent implantation is superior to balloon angioplasty for chronic coronary occlusions: six-year clinical follow-up of the GISSOC trial. J Am Coll Cardiol 2003; 41(9): 1488–92

18. Rubartelli P, Niccoli L, Verna E et al. Stent implantation versus balloon angioplasty in chronic coronary occlusions: results from the GISSOC trial. Gruppo Italiano di Studio sullo Stent nelle Occlusioni Coronariche. J Am Coll Cardiol 1998; 32(1): 90–96

19. Weaver WD, Simes RJ, Betriu A et al. Comparison of primary coronary angioplasty and intravenous thrombolytic therapy for acute myocardial infarction: a quantitative review. JAMA 1997; 278(23): 2093–98

20. Zijlstra F, Hoorntje JC, de Boer MJ et al. Long-term benefit of primary angioplasty as compared with thrombolytic therapy for acute myocardial infarction. N Engl J Med 1999; 341(19): 1413–19

21. Grines CL, Cox DA, Stone GW et al. Coronary angioplasty with or without stent implantation for acute myocardial infarction. Stent Primary Angioplasty in Myocardial Infarction Study Group. N Engl J Med 1999; 341(26): 1949–56

22. Stone GW, Grines CL, Cox DA et al. Comparison of angioplasty with stenting, with or without abciximab, in acute myocardial infarction. N Engl J Med 2002; 346(13): 957–66.

# PART III

# CLINICAL EXPERIENCE WITH DRUG-ELUTING STENTS

# 7. CLINICAL TRIALS: BARE METAL STENTS VERSUS DRUG-ELUTING STENTS

## Ali F Aboufares and Stephen R Ramee

## Background

Coronary stent implantation is associated with a significantly reduced restenosis rate compared to balloon angioplasty.[1,2] Stents achieve this benefit by eliminating elastic recoil and preventing negative vascular remodeling.[3,4] However, in-stent restenosis (ISR) due to neointimal hyperplasia remains a significant problem. During the past decade, numerous systemic pharmacologic and device-based therapies tried have failed to reduce the rate of ISR.[5] Recently, the delivery of antiproliferative or immunosuppressive drugs has shown promising results in inhibiting neointimal hyperplasia (Table 7.1).

**Table 7.1. Pivotal randomized drug-eluting stent versus bare metal stent trials for de-novo coronary artery stenosis**

| Study | n (patients) | RVD (mm) | Lesion length (mm) | Follow-up (months) | BS (%) | P value | Stent thrombosis |
|---|---|---|---|---|---|---|---|
| RAVEL[11] (sirolimus) | 238 | 2.6 | 9.6 | 6 | SES 0% BMS 26.6% | P < 0.001 | 0% |
| SIRIUS[12] (sirolimus) | 1058 | 2.5–3.5 | 15–30 | 8 | SES 3.2% BMS 35.4% | P < 0.001 | BMS 0.8% SES 0.4% |
| TAXUS II[14] (paclitaxel) | 536 | 2.75 | 10.5 | 12 | SR 2.3% MR 4.7% BMS 17.9% | P < 0.001 P = 0.002 | 0% |
| TAXUS IV[16] (paclitaxel) | 1314 | 2.5–3.75 | 10–28 | 9 | PES 7.9% BMS 26.6% | P < 0.001 | BMS 0.8% PES 0.6% |
| ASPECT[17] (paclitaxel) | 177 | 2.25-3.5 | <15 | 6 | LD 12% HD 4% BMS 27% | P < 0.001 | BMS 0% PES 0.03% |
| ELUTES[18] (paclitaxel) | 192 | 2.96 | <15 | 6 | PES (µg/mm$^2$): 0.2 µg/mm$^2$ 20% 0.7 µg/mm$^2$ 14% 1.4 µg/mm$^2$ 13% 2.7 µg/mm$^2$ 3% BMS 20.6% | P = 0.056 | 0% |

BS, binary stenosis; HD, high-dose PES (3.1 µg/mm$^2$); LD, low-dose PES (1.3 µg/mm$^2$); MR, moderate-release PES; PES, paclitaxel-eluting stent; RVD, reference vessel diameter; SES, sirolimus-eluting stent; SR, slow-release PES.

## Sirolimus

The first clinical experience with sirolimus followed extensive animal trials[6–8] and was a study that compared two different formulations: fast (100% of drug released in the first 15 days) versus slow release (20% of drug released in the first 15 days). A total of 45 patients with angina pectoris underwent elective percutaneous coronary intervention (PCI) with either the fast release (30 patients) or the slow release formulation (15 patients). A two-year angiographic and intravascular ultrasound (IVUS) follow-up demonstrated unchanged in-stent lumen dimensions, i.e. no evidence of occlusive intimal hyperplasia. Angiographic lumen loss, however, was higher in the fast-release group (0.28 vs 0.09 mm; P = 0.007).[9]

These early promising results paved the way for a study that evaluated the efficacy of the sirolimus-eluting stent in a placebo-controlled randomized trial (RAVEL: RAndomized, double-blind study with the sirolimus-eluting Bx VElocity™ balloon-expandable stent in the treatment of patients with de-novo native coronary artery Lesions). A total of 238 patients with discrete (type A), short (mean lesion length 9.6 mm), de-novo lesions were randomized to stenting with either the sirolimus-eluting stent (SES; $n$ = 120) or the bare metal stent group (BMS; $n$ = 118 patients). The mean reference diameter was 2.6 mm. The mean late loss at six months in the SES group was 0.01 mm versus 0.80 mm in the BMS control group (P < 0.001) (Table 7.2). The binary restenosis rate (> 50% luminal diameter) was 0% with the SES group versus 26.6% for the BMS control group (P < 0.001). There were no episodes of stent thrombosis.

A subgroup analysis showed that SES was highly effective in diabetic patients where the late loss was 0.08 mm and the restenosis rate was 0% compared to 0.82 mm and 42% respectively, in the BMS control group. At

**Table 7.2. RAVEL: six-month quantitative angiography.[11]**

|  | Sirolimus | Control n = 120 | P value n = 118 |
|---|---|---|---|
| Lesion length (mm) | 9.56 | 9.61 | NS |
| Reference diameter (mm) | 2.60 | 2.64 | NS |
| MLD pre (mm) | 0.94 | 0.95 | NS |
| MLD post (mm) | 2.43 | 2.41 | NS |
| MLD F/U (mm) | 2.42 | 1.64 | <0.001 |
| Late loss (mm) | −0.01 | 0.80 | <0.001 |
| Restenosis (%) | 0 | 26.6 | <0.001 |

F/U, follow-up; MLD, minimal lumen diameter; NS, non-significant.

one year, the investigators reported an overall rate of major adverse cardiac events (MACE) of 5.8% in the SES group and 28.8% in the BMS group (P < 0.001). This was mainly due to a higher rate of target vessel revascularization (TVR) in the BMS control group.

A subgroup analysis (n = 95 patients) using IVUS demonstrated nearly complete inhibition of the neointimal formation in the SES group. Incomplete stent apposition in the SES group (21%) was higher than in the BMS control group (4%) (Figure 7.1).[10] This phenomenon was not associated with adverse clinical events.[11]

The SIRIUS trial (SIRollmUS-coated Bx Velocity stent) was the pivotal study for the safety and efficacy of the SES (slow-release formulation) in more complex coronary lesions; long lesions (15–30 mm; mean 14.4 mm), small reference diameter (2.5–3.5 mm, mean 2.8 mm) and diabetics (26%). A total of 1058 patients were randomly assigned in a double-blind fashion to either the SES or the BMS control groups. Eight-month angiographic follow-up was achieved in 85% of patients including a subset with preplanned IVUS analysis.

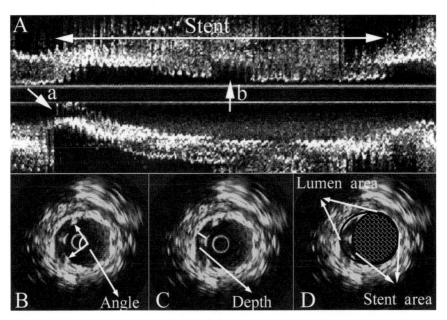

**Figure 7.1:** Methodology used to evaluate incomplete apposition at follow-up by IVUS. The figures illustrate the variety of measurements performed to quantify the incomplete apposition observed. (a) Location of incomplete apposition (arrows 'a' and 'b') on a longitudinal view. (b) Circumferential extent in angular degree. (c) Maximal depth (distance between the vessel wall and the most incompletely apposed strut. (d) Area of incomplete apposition (lumen area – stent area = incomplete apposition area) in a single IVUS cross-section (Reproduced with permission from reference 10.)

The binary in-stent restenosis (ISR) rate in patients with the SES was 3.2% versus 35.4% in the BMS control group (P < 0.001) (Figures 7.2 and 7.3). However, the in-segment analysis (including 5.0 mm proximal and distal to the stent margins) revealed a binary restenosis rate in the SES group of 8.9% versus 36.3% in the BMS control group (P < 0.001). This 'edge effect' was more pronounced in the proximal segment and was attributed to the stents not covering the entire region of balloon injury. This phenomenon did not translate into any worse clinical outcomes. Target vessel failure (TVF) was significantly lower in the SES group (8.6% vs 21.0%; P < 0.001) (Figure 7.4).

Adverse clinical outcomes were comparable in both groups with similar rates of death (0.9% in SES group vs 0.6% in the BMS control group) and MI (2.8% vs 3.2%, respectively). The cumulative frequency of stent thrombosis was 0.4% in the SES group versus 0.8% in the BMS control group, thus establishing the safety of the SES in this cohort of patients.

Despite the aforementioned safety and efficacy profile, certain subsets of patients (e.g. insulin-dependent diabetics) had a binary restenosis of about 35% with a late loss of 0.59 mm in the SES group (not statistically different from the BMS control group). This represents an example of unresolved challenging situations, i.e. small vessels, bifurcation lesions, SVG interventions, and ISR.

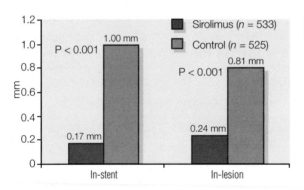

Figure 7.2: The SIRIUS trial: late loss analysis.[12]

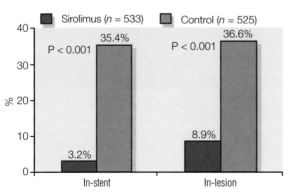

Figure 7.3: The SIRIUS trial: restenosis.[12]

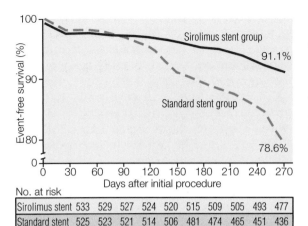

Figure 7.4: Actuarial rate of survival free from target-vessel failure among patients who received either a sirolimus-eluting stent or a standard stent. (Reproduced with permission from Moses JW, Leon MB, Popma JJ et al. Sirolimus-eluting stents versus standard stents in patients with stenosis in a native coronary artery. N Engl J Med 2003; 349(14): 1315–23.[12]

## Paclitaxel

As described earlier, paclitaxel-coated stents have shown promise in limiting restenosis in animal studies. Clinical trials were conducted to test various stent designs, dose densities, and release formulations with or without a polymer carrier. The TAXUS I trial (61 patients, with de-novo coronary lesions up to 12 mm long and 3.0 mm in diameter undergoing stent implantation, were randomized to paclitaxel-coated or bare NIRx™ Conformer stent) demonstrated safety of the stent and reported a reduction of restenosis from 11% to 0% after six months. The results of the study continued to demonstrate efficacy at 12 months.[13]

TAXUS I tested a slow-release formulation, while TAXUS II evaluated the performance of both slow-release (SR) and moderate-release (MR) polymers. A total of 536 patients were randomized to a SR paclitaxel-coated stent versus control or MR versus control. The mean reference vessel diameter was about 2.75 mm among the three groups and the mean lesion length was 10.5 mm. The 12-month target lesion revascularization was 14.4% in the combined BMS control group, 4.7% in the SR, and 3.8% in the MR group. Binary restenosis in the stented segment was 17.9% in the combined BMS control group, 2.3% in the SR, and 4.7% for MR. In both the SR and MR arms, there were no occurrences of late thrombosis.[14]

TAXUS III examined the feasibility of implanting up to two paclitaxel-coated stents for the treatment of ISR. The study was a single arm, small registry of 30 patients with ISR less than 30 mm in length, using the SR formulation. At six months, MACE were 29% with a TLR of about 21%, mostly attributed to geographic miss. In addition, no stent thrombosis was reported at up to 12 months.[15]

The pivotal study that led to the FDA approval of the paclitaxel-coated stents was the TAXUS IV trial, a prospective, randomized, double-blind study. A total of 1314 patients with de-novo lesions (vessel diameter 2.5–3.75 mm; lesion length 10–28 mm) were randomly assigned to either a BMS or an identical-appearing, SR, polymer-based, paclitaxel-eluting stent. Diabetes mellitus was present in 24.2% of the sample. A nine-month follow-up disclosed an impressive reduction in restenosis from 26.6% in the BMS group to 7.9% in the paclitaxel-eluting stent group (see Figure 7.5). Similarly, a reduction from 12.0% to 4.7% was noted in TVR. Stent thrombosis and MACE were not different between the two groups.[16]

In contrast to polymer-based paclitaxel-coated stents, a technique of stent surface modification to make paclitaxel adhere to the outer or abluminal surface of the stent has been developed. ASPECT and ELUTES were two trials to evaluate non-polymeric paclitaxel-eluting stent in various doses. ASPECT (ASian Paclitaxel-Eluting stent Clinical Trial) randomized 177 patients into three different arms: high-dose ($3.10 \mu g/mm^2$), low dose ($1.28 \mu g/mm^2$) paclitaxel; or a bare metal Supra G™ stent (Cook, Inc., Bloomington, IN) with a single, de-novo, native coronary lesion with a diameter of 2.25 to 3.5 mm. Six-month follow-up revealed a dose-dependent binary restenosis rate ranging from 27% for BMS, to 12% for the low-dose, and a 4% for the high-dose group (Figure 7.6). No subacute stent thrombosis was noted in the aspirin and clopidogrel/ticlopidine, however 15% of patients who had aspirin and cilostazol as the antiplatelet regimen had subacute stent thrombosis (all of which had the drug-coated stent).[17]

ELUTES (European EvaLUation of pacliTaxel-Eluting Stent) used the V-Flex Plus™ stent (Cook, Inc., Bloomington, IN) in 192 patients with single, de-novo, coronary lesions randomized to either BMS or one of four paclitaxel dose densities (0.2, 0.7, 1.4, or $2.7 \mu g/mm^2$) paclitaxel loaded onto the stent without any polymer. At six months, the corresponding binary restenosis rate was 21% in the BMS group, and 20%, 12%, 14%, and 3%, respectively

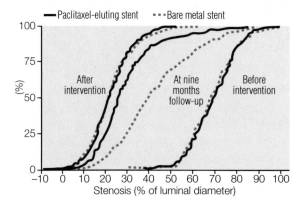

Figure 7.5: Cumulative distribution curves (paired-lesion analysis) for percent stenosis of the luminal diameter in the group that received a paclitaxel-eluting stent and the group that received a bare metal stent before and immediately after the intervention and at nine months. (Reproduced with permission from reference 16.)

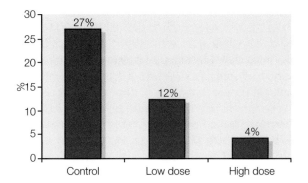

Figure 7.6: ASPECT trial results. Paclitaxel at low versus high dose.[17]

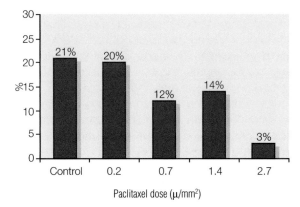

Figure 7.7: ELUTES trial: restenosis rates.[18]

Paclitaxel dose ($\mu$/mm$^2$)

(between control and high-dose paclitaxel; P = 0.056) (Figure 7.7). No stent thrombosis occurred confirming safety as well as efficacy for this stent. The study demonstrated a near-linear relationship between efficacy and dosage with the minimal effective paclitaxel dose being 2.7 µg/mm$^2$.[18]

Recently published data utilizing everolimus, an antiproliferative agent similar in action to sirolimus, showed promising initial results. FUTURE I (First Use To Underscore restenosis Reduction with Everolimus) trial is a prospective single-blind trial that randomized 42 patients with de-novo coronary lesions into everolimus-eluting stent (EES) versus BMS. Six-month angiographic restenosis was 0% in the EES versus 9.1% (one patient) in the BMS group (P = NS) with no late stent thrombosis, thus demonstrating safety and efficacy in this initial clinical experience.[19]

## Failed trials

The SCORE (Study to COmpare REstenosis rate between QueST and QuaDDS-QP2) trial randomized 266 patients to either the QuaDDS-QP2 DES or the QueST (bare metal) stent (Figure 7.8). The QuaDDS-QP2 stent (Quanam Medical Corp., Santa Clara, CA; Boston Scientific, Natick, MA) is a stainless steel stent with polymer sleeves that elute QP2 (7-hexanoyltaxol, a taxane analog) in a controlled fashion. Preliminary human studies showed that local delivery of 7-hexanoyltaxol (a taxol-derived lipophilic microtubule inhibitor-QP2) reduced neointimal growth after PCI.[20] The study was halted because of an unacceptable late thrombosis rate at one year (Figure 7.9).[21,22]

The DELIVER trial (Non-Polymer-Based Paclitaxel-Coated Coronary Stents for the Treatment of Patients With De-Novo Coronary Lesions) was a prospective, randomized, blinded, multicenter clinical evaluation of the non-polymer-based paclitaxel-coated ACHIEVE™ stent (Cook, Inc., Bloomington, IN) compared with the stainless steel Multi-Link PENTA™ stent (Guidant Corp., Indianapolis, IN). A total of 1043 patients with focal, de-novo, coronary lesions, less than 25 mm in length, and 2.5- to 4.0-mm vessels were randomized. Eight-month angiographic follow-up depicted a reduction of in-stent binary restenosis which did not meet statistical significance (14.9% vs 20.6% for the BMS; P = 0.076) (Figure 7.10). Target vessel failure for the ACHIEVE™ stent group was 11.9% versus 14.5% for control (P = 0.12) thereby not meeting its projected end-point of 40% reduction in TVF.[23]

The ACTION trial (Actinomycin-eluting stent for coronary revascularization: a randomized feasibility and safety study) tested a different antiproliferative agent, Actinomycin-D. A total of 360 patients were randomized to either a 10 μg/mm² Actinomycin-D-loaded Multi-Link TETRA-D™ stent, a 2.5 μg/mm² loaded stent, or a bare metal Multi-Link TETRA-D™ stent. The trial was prematurely terminated because of the absence of any benefit at six

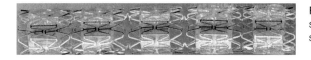

Figure 7.8: The QuaDDS stent with five polymer sleeves.

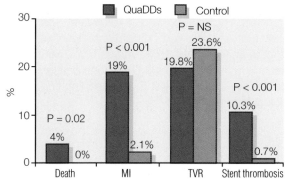

Figure 7.9: SCORE trial. One-year cumulative major adverse coronary event and stent thrombosis. MI, myocardial infarction; NS, non-significant; TVR, target vessel revascularization.[22]

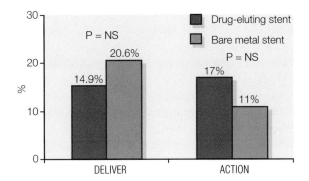

months. The binary restenosis rate was 17% for the high dose, 25% for the low dose, and 11% for the BMS (see Figure 7.10). Failure was attributed to the 'edge effect' phenomenon.[24]

## Conclusion

The local delivery of antiproliferative or immunosuppressive drugs using stents has shown promising results in inhibiting neointimal hyperplasia. Efficacy of DES in animal models does not always yield similar results in humans. Trials with various formulations of paclitaxel demonstrate the importance of dosimetry and stent design in order to produce a successful DES. At the present time, only two DES have proven effective in large randomized trials: Cypher (Cordis, Miami, FL) a sirolimus-eluting stent and Taxus (BSC, Watertown, MA) polymer-based paclitaxel-eluting stents. Differences in outcomes between DES may be due to treating different lesion subsets. Late thrombosis and aneurysm formation have not been associated with the use of sirolimus-eluting stents so far. The high incidence of stent thrombosis observed in the SCORE trial remind us that the safety of these stents must be carefully assessed.

## References

1. Serruys PW, de Jaegere P, Kiemeneij F et al. A comparison of balloon-expandable stent implantation with balloon angioplasty in patients with coronary artery disease. Benestent Study Group. N Engl J Med 1994; 331(8): 489–95

2. Fischman DL, Leon MB, Baim DS et al. A randomized comparison of coronary-stent placement and balloon angioplasty in the treatment of coronary artery disease. Stent Restenosis Study Investigators. N Engl J Med 1994; 331(8): 496–501

3. Lafont A, Guzman LA, Whitlow PL et al. Restenosis after experimental angioplasty. Intimal, medial, and adventitial changes associated with constrictive remodeling. Circ Res 1995; 76(6): 996–1002

4. Mintz GS, Popma JJ, Pichard AD et al. Arterial remodeling after coronary angioplasty: a serial intravascular ultrasound study. Circulation 1996; 94(1): 35–43

5. Hoffmann R, Mintz GS. Coronary in-stent restenosis – predictors, treatment and prevention. Eur Heart J 2000; 21(21): 1739–49

6. Gallo R, Padurean A, Jayaraman T et al. Inhibition of intimal thickening after balloon angioplasty in porcine coronary arteries by targeting regulators of the cell cycle. Circulation 1999; 99(16): 2164–70

7. Suzuki T, Kopia G, Hayashi S et al. Stent-based delivery of sirolimus reduces neointimal formation in a porcine coronary model. Circulation 2001; 104(10): 1188–93

8. Klugherz BD, Llanos G, Lieuallen W et al. Twenty-eight-day efficacy and pharmacokinetics of the sirolimus-eluting stent. Coron Artery Dis 2002; 13(3): 183–88

9. Sousa JE, Costa MA, Sousa AG et al. Two-year angiographic and intravascular ultrasound follow-up after implantation of sirolimus-eluting stents in human coronary arteries. Circulation 2003; 107(3): 381–83

10. Serruys PW, Degertekin M, Tanabe K et al. Intravascular ultrasound findings in the multicenter, randomized, double-blind RAVEL (RAndomized study with the sirolimus-eluting VElocity balloon-expandable stent in the treatment of patients with de novo native coronary artery Lesions) trial. Circulation 2002; 106(7): 798–803

11. Regar E, Serruys PW, Bode C et al. Angiographic findings of the multicenter Randomized Study With the Sirolimus-Eluting Bx VELOCITY™ Balloon-Expandable Stent (RAVEL): sirolimus-eluting stents inhibit restenosis irrespective of the vessel size. Circulation 2002; 106(15): 1949–56

12. Moses JW, Leon MB, Popma JJ et al. Sirolimus-eluting stents versus standard stents in patients with stenosis in a native coronary artery. N Engl J Med 2003; 349(14): 1315–23

13. Grube E, Silber S, Hauptmann KE et al. TAXUS I: six- and twelve-month results from a randomized, double-blind trial on a slow-release paclitaxel-eluting stent for de novo coronary lesions. Circulation 2003; 107(1): 38–42

14. Colombo A, Drzewiecki J, Banning A et al. Randomized study to assess the effectiveness of slow- and moderate-release polymer-based paclitaxel-eluting stents for coronary artery lesions. Circulation 2003; 108(7): 788–94

15. Tanabe K, Serruys PW, Grube E et al. TAXUS III Trial: in-stent restenosis treated with stent-based delivery of paclitaxel incorporated in a slow-release polymer formulation. Circulation 2003; 107(4): 559–64

16. Stone GW, Ellis SG, Cox DA et al. A polymer-based, paclitaxel-eluting stent in patients with coronary artery disease. N Engl J Med 2004; 350(3): 221–31

17. Park SJ, Shim WH, Ho DS et al. A paclitaxel-eluting stent for the prevention of coronary restenosis. N Engl J Med 2003; 348(16): 1537–45

18. Gershlick A, De Scheerder I, Chevalier B et al. Inhibition of restenosis with a paclitaxel-eluting, polymer-free coronary stent: the European evaLUation of pacliTaxel Eluting Stent (ELUTES) trial. Circulation 2004; 109(4): 487–93

19. Grube E, Sonoda S, Ikeno F et al. Six- and twelve-month results from first human experience using everolimus-eluting stents with bioabsorbable polymer. Circulation 2004; 109(18): 2168–71

20. De la Fuente LM, Miano J, Mrad J et al. Initial results of the Quanam drug-eluting stent (QuaDS-QP-2) Registry (BARDDS) in human subjects. Catheter Cardiovasc Interv 2001; 53(4): 480–88

21. Kataoka T, Grube E, Honda Y et al. 7-Hexanoyltaxol-eluting stent for prevention of neointimal growth: an intravascular ultrasound analysis from the Study to COmpare REstenosis rate between QueST and QuaDS-QP2 (SCORE). Circulation 2002; 106(14): 1788–93

22. Grube E, Lansky A, Hauptmann KE et al. High-dose 7-hexanoyltaxol-eluting stent with polymer sleeves for coronary revascularization: one-year results from the SCORE randomized trial. J Am Coll Cardiol 2004; 44(7): 1368–72

23. Lansky AJ, Costa RA, Mintz GS et al. Non-polymer-based paclitaxel-coated coronary stents for the treatment of patients with de novo coronary lesions: angiographic follow-up of the DELIVER clinical trial. Circulation 2004; 109(16): 1948–54

24. Serruys PW, Ormiston JA, Sianos G et al. Actinomycin-eluting stent for coronary revascularization: a randomized feasibility and safety study: the ACTION trial. J Am Coll Cardiol 2004; 44(7): 1363–67

# 8. BROADER INDICATIONS (OFF-LABEL USE) FOR CORONARY DRUG-ELUTING STENTS

## Albert W Chan

## Introduction

In the USA, the drug-eluting stents (DES) (Cypher: Cordis, Miami, FL; and Taxus: Boston Scientific, Inc., Maple Ridge, MN) were approved by the Food and Drug Administration (FDA) for clinical use according to the same clinical and anatomical criteria that were used in the pivotal pre-approval trials (SIRIUS and TAXUS IV) (Box 8.1).[1,2] However, over 50% of the patients in our clinical practice would not fit into these criteria.[3,4]

Box 8.1 Major exclusion criteria in the DES pre-approval clinical trials

Clinical characteristics
- Age <18 or >80 years
- Acute or recent (<48 hours) MI including non-ST elevation MI
- Left ventricular ejection fraction <30%
- Unable to tolerate aspirin or ADP-receptor antagonist
- Serum creatinine >2.0 mg/dl

Anatomical characteristics
- Left main coronary artery lesion
- Target lesion within bypass graft
- Reference diameter <2.5 mm or >3.5 mm
- Lesion length <10 or >28 mm
- Angulated lesion (>60°)
- Bifurcation lesion or side-branch involvement
- Post-angioplasty restenosis or in-stent restenosis
- Ostial lesion
- Concomitant use of brachytherapy

Since the introduction of stents more than a decade ago, primary stent placement has become the standard strategy for a very broad range of clinical and anatomical indications, e.g. stable and unstable syndromes, or acute myocardial infarction (MI), complex coronary lesions, left main stenosis, and bypass graft. The long-term patency of stents has been limited by restenosis until the availability of the DES. Accordingly, it is logical to consider expanding the indications of DES beyond those that were studied in the clinical trials.

Indeed, Lemos and colleagues have reported the outcomes of unrestricted use of sirolimus-eluting stents in a 'real world' setting.[5] This study compared the outcomes of 450 consecutive percutaneous coronary intervention (PCI) patients before (2.5–3.0 mm bare metal stents, BMS) and 508 consecutive PCI patients (2.5–3.0 mm Cypher™ stents) following the approval of Cypher™ stents in Europe. The study concluded that, during the 12 months of follow-up, the risk of death or MI was not different between DES and BMS groups, and the risk of target vessel revascularization (TVR) was significantly lower in the DES group (3.7% vs 10.9%; P < 0.001).

Shortly after the initial launch of the Cypher™ stents in the USA, the FDA published a physician alert about reports of subacute stent thrombosis including 60 fatal events.[6] The etiology of these events was unknown. Localized vascular hypersensitivity reaction to the polymer coating (poly-*n*-butyl methacrylate and polyethylene-vinyl acetate copolymer) on the Cypher™ stent causing late thrombosis has been proposed.[7] Alternatively, this could be in part explained by stent malapposition due to the limited availability of various sizes of the Cypher™ stent shortly after the stent approval, though this remains purely speculative. In post-market surveillance, the incidence of acute stent thrombosis did not appear to be higher than that reported in the historical controls,[8] provided that the sizes of the vessels and the stents were well matched and complete coverage of the lesions was made. Moreover, subsequent clinical trials as well as our clinical practice have extended the administration of clopidogrel to 3–6 months from the traditional 30-day period to improve the protection against subacute stent thrombosis.

## Off-label indications for drug-eluting stents

### Acute coronary syndromes

Coronary lesions associated with acute coronary syndromes (ACS) – including ST-elevation MI (STEMI), non-STEMI, and unstable angina – differ from stable coronary artery lesions in that the former are more thrombogenic and have a greater number of inflammatory cells. In a series of 198 consecutive patients undergoing DES implantation for ACS,[9] the incidence of death, MI, or target lesion revascularization (TLR) at 30 days was not different from the historical controls who received various brands of BMS (6.1% vs 6.6%; P = 0.85). In particular, the risk of subacute stent thrombosis was not different (0.5% vs 1.7%; P = 0.41).

In another report which included 186 consecutive patients with acute STEMI patients, and who received DES during primary intervention,[10] the incidence of major adverse coronary events (MACE) was significantly lower when compared with the historical controls (Table 8.1); the benefit was predominantly due to less reintervention. Stent thrombosis was not present

Table 8.1. Adverse events in patients with acute MI undergoing primary intervention with DES [9]

|  | DES (n = 186) | BMS (n = 183) | P |
|---|---|---|---|
| **30-day events** |  |  |  |
| Death | 5.9% | 5.5% | NS |
| Death or non-fatal MI | 6.5% | 7.1% | NS |
| Target vessel revascularization | 1.1% | 4.4% | NS |
| Stent thrombosis | 0% | 1.6% | 0.1 |
| **300-day events** |  |  |  |
| Death | 8.3% | 8.2% | NS |
| Death or non-fatal MI | 8.8% | 10.4% | NS |
| Target vessel revascularization | 1.1% | 8.2% | <0.01 |

within the first 30 days. Of note, the duration of clopidogrel administration was longer in the DES group than the control group ($3.7 \pm 2.1$ vs $2.1 \pm 1.5$ months; $P < 0.01$), and this might explain the lower incidence of subacute stent thrombosis events.[8] These observations in large registries confirm the safety and the durability of DES in the setting of ACS including STEMI.

## Bifurcation lesions

Bifurcation lesions have traditionally posed a serious challenge to interventional cardiologists. Various techniques have been developed to treat bifurcation lesions (Figure 8.1) but no single technique has been superior to another. Using DES, Colombo and colleagues[11] demonstrated the feasibility of the crushed stent technique (or modified T-stent technique). In the RESEARCH registry,[12] bifurcation stenting with DES was associated with an increased risk of restenosis by univariate analysis, but this did not appear to be a factor after adjusting for ostial location and vessel diameter. In a randomized trial which included 91 patients undergoing DES placement in bifurcation lesions, the six-month clinical outcomes were similar when both vessels had stents placed (T-stent) or when only stenting the parent vessel (Table 8.2).[13]

Table 8.2. Comparison of T-stent versus stenting of the parent vessel alone in bifurcating lesions using DES stents[13]

| Six-month events | T-stent (n = 44) | Stent parent vessel only (n = 47) |
|---|---|---|
| Death | 2 | 0 |
| MI | 0 | 4 |
| TVR | 5 | 2 |
| Death, MI, or TVR | 7 | 6 |

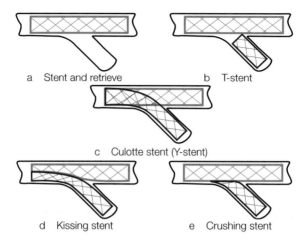

a   Stent and retrieve    b   T-stent

c   Culotte stent (Y-stent)

d   Kissing stent    e   Crushing stent

**Figure 8.1:** Techniques of bifurcation stent placement with side-branch (the upper arm in each diagram represents the parent vessel): (a) In the stent and retrieve method a stent is placed in the parent vessel after optimization of the ostium of the side-branch with balloon angioplasty. If the sidebranch is compromised after parent vessel stenting, balloon angioplasty and provisional stenting is performed after recrossing the stent strut. (b) In the T-stent method a stent is intentionally placed in the side-branch and the balloon catheter and the guidewire are then withdrawn from the side-branch, followed by stenting of the parent vessel. (c) In the culotte stent technique the parent vessel and the side-branch are stented sequentially with overlapping in the parent vessel. The parent vessel is then rewired through the stent strut and kissing balloon inflation is performed to optimize the outcome. This is used particularly in bifurcations where the angle between the two branches is small. (d) In the kissing stent technique the two stents are deployed simultaneously. This technique is used when there is a diameter mismatch between the proximal vessel and the two branches. (e) In the crushing stent technique the two DES stents are delivered to the bifurcating lesion, with part of the proximal portion (~5 mm) of the side-branch stent left within the parent vessel after its deployment. The side-branch balloon and guidewire are then removed, followed by stent deployment in the parent vessel. At the discretion of the operator, kissing balloon angioplasty may be performed to optimize the angiographic result.

Considering the cost of DES, stenting of the parent vessel combined with angioplasty and provisional stenting for the side-branch is probably the preferable technique for the treatment of the bifurcation lesions since this appears to be as effective as routinely placing a stent in the side-branch.

## Unprotected left main

In the bare stent era, left main coronary stenting was limited to several specific high-risk settings (Box 8.2).[5] In the largest left main stent registry (ULTIMA),[14,15] poor left ventricular ejection fraction (<30%), severe mitral regurgitation, cardiogenic shock, moderate or severe renal insufficiency (serum creatinine >2.0 mg/dl), and severe lesion calcification were independent risk factors for mortality at nine months after unprotected left main coronary stenting. The outcomes for low-risk patients (i.e. age <65 years, left ventricular ejection fraction >30%, and no cardiogenic shock) appeared to be acceptable (one year: mortality 3.4%; MI 2.3%; bypass surgery rate 11.3%). Large reference diameter and non-distal left main lesions were also associated with favorable outcomes with left main stenting.[16–18]

---

**Box 8.2 Specific clinical settings when coronary stenting may be preferable to bypass surgery**

- High surgical risk:
  - medical comorbidity, e.g. severe chronic obstructive lung disease
  - extreme elderly
  - multiple prior cardiac bypass surgeries
  - chest irradiation
  - acute MI
  - left ventricular systolic function <20%
- Poor distal target for bypass surgery
- No bypassable left anterior descending or circumflex artery

---

In a consecutive series of unprotected left main lesions treated with DES, restenosis was reported in 19% of patients and it occurred solely in lesions involving the distal left main bifurcation (Table 8.3).[19] In another series, DES for elective left main revascularization was associated with a favorable outcome; in particular there were no adverse events within the first five months after discharge.[20] Therefore, when a correctly sized DES is available, unprotected left main stenting appears to be feasible but a larger series of patients will be necessary to judge the safety and efficacy of this treatment for elective indications (Figure 8.2). Distal left main stenting is feasible but restenosis rates remain high in this location despite the use of DES. The role of intravascular ultrasound IVUS remains to be determined in this group of patients.

**Table 8.3. Outcomes of unprotected left main stent placement ($n$ = 32) with DES[19]**

|  | Death | MI | TLR |
|---|---|---|---|
| In-hospital | 0 | 0 | 1 |
| 6 months | 1 | 1 | 6 |

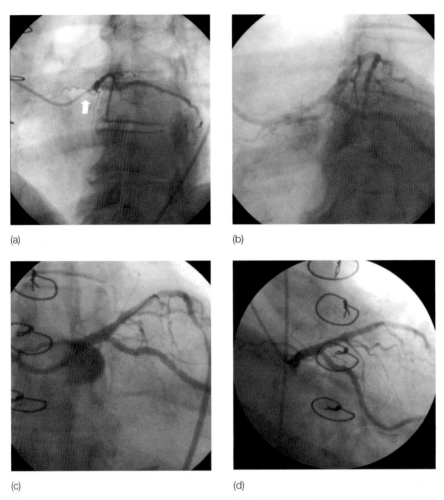

(a)

(b)

(c)

(d)

Figure 8.2: This 59-year-old female patient was referred because of recurrent angina within a week after coronary bypass surgery for a left main coronary artery stenosis. Repeat angiography revealed that all the bypass grafts were occluded. (a) Percutaneous coronary intervention of the left main coronary artery (LMCA) was considered (arrow). (b) Using a 6F left Judkins guiding catheter, balloon dilation with a 2.5 × 15 mm balloon was performed and a Taxus 3.5 × 13 mm stent was positioned in the LMCA. (c) Immediate result after stent deployment. (d) Follow-up angiogram at three months.

## In-stent restenosis and brachytherapy failures

Vascular brachytherapy has been the preferred treatment for in-stent restenosis (ISR).[21–29] The therapeutic effect of brachytherapy is related to the cytostatic effect of the electromagnetic energy, causing breakdown of the single- and double-stranded DNA in actively dividing cells. The efficacy of brachytherapy is balanced by late restenosis and late thrombosis, and the fact that delivery of brachytherapy in the catheterization laboratory is associated with a number of logistical issues, e.g. radiation oncologists and physicists are not readily available in many institutions.

Local delivery of antiproliferative drugs using a stent platform is an attractive alternative for the treatment of ISR. It may obviate the need for other personnel to administer radiation treatment. Sousa and colleagues demonstrated the feasibility of using DES to treat ISR in 25 patients.[30] In the other studies,[31,32] the use of DES for the treatment of ISR or lesions after brachytherapy failure is feasible, but the results are less impressive when compared to those obtained in de-novo lesions (Table 8.4). The feasibility of a paclitaxel-eluting stent for ISR was shown in the TAXUS III study in which 28 patients with ISR were treated (see Table 8.4).[33] During follow-up, eight patients (29%) had MACE (one post-procedural non-Q-wave MI, one coronary bypass surgery for left main disease remote from the target lesion, and six TLR including three with malapposition of stent struts by IVUS assessment).

Factors to be considered when investigating the differences in the clinical response of ISR and de-novo lesions to DES include: pharmacokinetics of drug diffusion across scar tissue; tissue response to DES after brachytherapy compared to de-novo lesions; longer stents used to treat ISR lesions than those used in de-novo lesions; and incomplete DES expansion that could occur due to a pre-existing stent within the same lesion. TAXUS V ISR is an ongoing large clinical trial to assess the efficacy of DES for the treatment of ISR.

## Small (⩽2.5 mm) and Large (⩾3.5 mm) vessels

Small vessel diameter is an important predictor for restenosis.[34,35] While BMS provide significant benefits in medium to large vessels (⩾3.0 mm), the benefit of routine stent strategy in small (⩽2.5 mm) coronary arteries is more controversial.[36–42] Stenting in small coronary arteries is limited by the high restenosis rate due to a relatively limited acute gain immediately after stent implantation with an obligatory late loss which results in restenosis. Strategies that reduce late loss, including DES, would be expected to be useful in smaller vessels (Figure 8.3). In both the SIRIUS and TAXUS IV studies,[43,44]

| Table 8.4. Clinical outcomes with the use of DES in ISR or after brachytherapy failure | | | | | | |
|---|---|---|---|---|---|---|
| Study | n | Prior brachytherapy | Follow-up | Death | MI | TLR |
| TAXUS III[33] | 28 | No | 12 months | 0 | 1 | 6 |
| Saia[32] | 12 | Yes | 4.5 months | 1 | 0 | 4 |
| Degertekin[31] | 16 | Yes | 9 months | 2 | 1 | 1 |

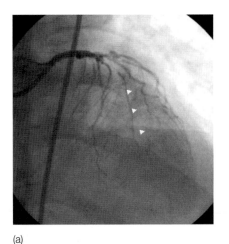

(a)

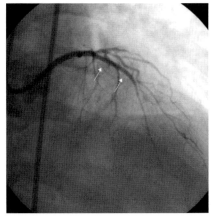

(b)

(c)

**Figure 8.3:** DES in a long lesion with small reference diameter (<2.5 mm). Percutaneous coronary intervention of a chronically occluded left anterior descending artery (LAD) was performed one week after a primary intervention of an inferior MI in a 72-year-old patient. (a) Baseline angiogram showed that the LAD was occluded. (b) Balloon dilation was performed followed by tandem stent placement using Cypher 2.5 × 18 mm and 2.5 × 23 mm stents (Cordis, Miami, FL) (arrows). (c) Repeat angiogram of the LAD (arrows) at five months.

vessel size of 2.50–2.75 mm was associated with an increase in restenosis rate when compared with large vessel sizes in both DES and BMS arms (Table 8.5), but the DES was superior to BMS in small vessels. Insight from the European registry in which 2.25 mm DES were used suggested that DES lowered the rate of TLR when compared with BMS (TLR at 12 months 5.5%, hazard ratio 0.33; P = 0.007).[5,45]

Large vessel interventions are associated with low risk of restenosis after stenting and hence the cost–benefit ratio of large vessel stenting with DES is expected to be lower than for small vessels. Despite that, in large vessels, DES yielded lower restenosis rates, with reported TLR of less than 4% at 12 months in the randomized trials (see Table 8.5).[43,44]

Recent registry data support the safety and feasibility of over-expanding DES with post-dilation with larger balloon catheters (1 mm greater than the

**Table 8.5. Target vessel revascularization at 12 months reported in the SIRIUS and TAXUS IV trials[1,43,44]**

| Vessel size | n | TLR (%) | |
|---|---|---|---|
| | | DES | Bare metal stent |
| **Cypher** | | | |
| <2.75 mm | 522 | 6.3 | 18.7 |
| ≥2.75 mm | 523 | 1.9 | 14.8 |
| **Taxus** | | | |
| ≤2.5 mm | 176 | 5.6 | 20.6 |
| >2.5 to <3.0 mm | 202 | 4.3 | 13.3 |
| ≥3.0 mm | 180 | 3.5 | 11.1 |

stent diameter at nominal pressure) in large vessels.[46] Concerns persist that insufficient local drug concentration may lead to inadequate inhibition of neointimal proliferation, as well as the potential risk of subacute thrombosis due to inadequate apposition of an undersized stent in a large vessel (e.g. a 3.5-mm DES implanted in a ≥ 4.0-mm vessel). Therefore, when the reference vessel diameter is larger than available DES, the use of a correctly sized BMS is recommended.

### Saphenous vein grafts

Stents were reported to lower the risk of restenosis in saphenous vein grafts (SVG) compared to balloon angioplasty in two non-randomized studies.[47,48] However, in a large randomized trial there was no benefit (37% vs 46%; $P = 0.24$).[49] Saphenous vein graft intervention remains as a major risk factor for death, MI, and restenosis.[50–55] Since intimal hyperplasia is the most important pathogenesis of ISR within SVG, it seems logical to use appropriately sized DES in SVG interventions, pending the demonstration of safety and efficacy of this lesion subgroup.

## References

1. Moses JW, Leon MB, Popma JJ et al. Sirolimus-eluting stents versus standard stents in patients with stenosis in a native coronary artery. N Engl J Med 2003; 349(14): 1315–23

2. Stone GW, Ellis SG, Cox DA et al. A polymer-based, paclitaxel-eluting stent in patients with coronary artery disease. N Engl J Med 2004; 350(3): 221–31

3. Klein LW, Block P, Brindis RG et al. Percutaneous coronary interventions in octogenarians in the American College of Cardiology – National Cardiovascular Data Registry: development of a nomogram predictive of in-hospital mortality. J Am Coll Cardiol 2002; 40(3): 394–402

4. Anderson HV, Shaw RE, Brindis RG et al. A contemporary overview of percutaneous coronary interventions. The American College of Cardiology – National Cardiovascular Data Registry (ACC–NCDR). J Am Coll Cardiol 2002; 39(7): 1096–103

5. Lemos PA, Serruys PW, van Domburg RT et al. Unrestricted utilization of sirolimus-eluting stents compared with conventional bare stent implantation in the "real world": the Rapamycin-Eluting Stent Evaluated At Rotterdam Cardiology Hospital (RESEARCH) registry. Circulation 2004; 109(2): 190–95

6. Curfman GD. Sirolimus-eluting coronary stents. N Engl J Med 2002; 346(23): 1770–71

7. Virmani R, Guagliumi G, Farb A et al. Localized hypersensitivity and late coronary thrombosis secondary to a sirolimus-eluting stent: should we be cautious? Circulation 2004; 109(6): 701–705

8. Jeremias A, Sylvia B, Bridges J et al. Stent thrombosis after successful sirolimus-eluting stent implantation. Circulation 2004; 109(16): 1930–32

9. Lemos PA, Lee CH, Degertekin M et al. Early outcome after sirolimus-eluting stent implantation in patients with acute coronary syndromes: insights from the Rapamycin-Eluting Stent Evaluated At Rotterdam Cardiology Hospital (RESEARCH) registry. J Am Coll Cardiol 2003; 41(11): 2093–99

10. Lemos PA, Saia F, Hofma SH et al. Short- and long-term clinical benefit of sirolimus-eluting stents compared to conventional bare stents for patients with acute myocardial infarction. J Am Coll Cardiol 2004; 43(4): 704–708

11. Colombo A, Stankovic G, Orlic D et al. Modified T-stenting technique with crushing for bifurcation lesions: immediate results and 30-day outcome. Catheter Cardiovasc Interv 2003; 60(2): 145–51

12. Lemos PA, Hoye A, Goedhart D et al. Clinical, angiographic, and procedural predictors of angiographic restenosis after sirolimus-eluting stent implantation in complex patients: an evaluation from the Rapamycin-Eluting Stent Evaluated At Rotterdam Cardiology Hospital (RESEARCH) study. Circulation 2004; 109(11): 1366–70

13. Pan M, Suarez de Lezo J, Pavlovic D et al. Drug-eluting stents for bifurcating coronary lesions: a randomized comparison of simple versus complex strategy approach. J Am Coll Cardiol 2004; 43: 87A

14. Ellis SG, Tamai H, Nobuyoshi M et al. Contemporary percutaneous treatment of unprotected left main coronary stenoses: initial results from a multicenter registry analysis 1994–1996. Circulation 1997; 96(11): 3867–72

15. Tan WA, Tamai H, Park SJ et al. Long-term clinical outcomes after unprotected left main trunk percutaneous revascularization in 279 patients. Circulation 2001; 104(14): 1609–14

16. Takagi T, Stankovic G, Finci L et al. Results and long-term predictors of adverse clinical events after elective percutaneous interventions on unprotected left main coronary artery. Circulation 2002; 106(6): 698–702

17. Park SJ, Hong MK, Lee CW et al. Elective stenting of unprotected left main coronary artery stenosis: effect of debulking before stenting and intravascular ultrasound guidance. J Am Coll Cardiol 2001; 38(4): 1054–60

18. McNamara T, Bomberger R, Merchant R. Intra-arterial urokinase as the initial therapy for acutely ischemic lower limbs. Circulation 2001; 83: 106

19. Chieffo A, Orlic D, Airoldi F et al. Early and mid-term results of Cypher stents in unprotected left main. J Am Coll Cardiol 2004; 43: 21A

20. Arampatzis CA, Lemos PA, Tanabe K et al. Effectiveness of sirolimus-eluting stent for treatment of left main coronary artery disease. Am J Cardiol 2003; 92(3): 327–29

21. Waksman R, Ajani AE, White RL et al. Intravascular gamma radiation for in-stent restenosis in saphenous-vein bypass grafts. N Engl J Med 2002; 346(16): 1194–99

22. Waksman R, Ajani AE, White RL et al. Four-year follow-up after intracoronary gamma-radiation therapy for in-stent restenosis: results from a randomized clinical trial. J Am Coll Cardiol 2002; 39: 64A

23. Waksman R, Raizner AE, Yeung AC et al. Use of localised intracoronary beta radiation in treatment of in-stent restenosis: the INHIBIT randomised controlled trial. Lancet 2002; 359(9306): 551–57

24. Waksman R, White RL, Chan RC et al. Intracoronary gamma-radiation therapy after angioplasty inhibits recurrence in patients with in-stent restenosis. Circulation 2000; 101(18): 2165–71

25. Teirstein PS, Massullo V, Jani S et al. Catheter-based radiotherapy to inhibit restenosis after coronary stenting. N Engl J Med 1997; 336(24): 1697–703

26. Teirstein PS, Massullo V, Jani S et al. Three-year clinical and angiographic follow-up after intracoronary radiation: results of a randomized clinical trial. Circulation 2000; 101(4): 360–65

27. Leon MB, Teirstein PS, Lansky AJ et al. Intracoronary gamma radiation to reduce in-stent restenosis: the multicenter GAMMA 1 randomized clinical trial. J Am Coll Cardiol 1999; 33: 19A

28. Leon MB, Teirstein PS, Moses J et al. Localized intracoronary gamma-radiation therapy to inhibit the recurrence of restenosis after stenting. N Engl J Med 2001; 344: 250–56

29. Popma JJ, Suntharalingham M, Lansky AJ et al. Randomized trial of 90Sr/90Y beta-radiation versus placebo control for treatment of in-stent restenosis. Circulation 2002; 106(9): 1090–96

30. Sousa JE, Costa MA, Abizaid A et al. Sirolimus-eluting stent for the treatment of in-stent restenosis: a quantitative coronary angiography and three-dimensional intravascular ultrasound study. Circulation 2003; 107(1): 24–27

31. Degertekin M, Regar E, Tanabe K et al. Sirolimus-eluting stent for treatment of complex in-stent restenosis: the first clinical experience. J Am Coll Cardiol 2003; 41(2): 184–89

32. Saia F, Lemos PA, Sianos G et al. Effectiveness of sirolimus-eluting stent implantation for recurrent in-stent restenosis after brachytherapy. Am J Cardiol 2003; 92(2): 200–203

33. Tanabe K, Serruys PW, Grube E et al. TAXUS III Trial: in-stent restenosis treated with stent-based delivery of paclitaxel incorporated in a slow-release polymer formulation. Circulation 2003; 107(4): 559–64

34. Foley DP, Melkert R, Serruys PW. Influence of coronary vessel size on renarrowing process and late angiographic outcome after successful balloon angioplasty. Circulation 1994; 90(3): 1239–51

35. Hirshfeld JW Jr, Schwartz JS, Hugo R et al. Restenosis after coronary angioplasty: a multivariate statistical model to relate lesion and procedure variables to restenosis. The M-HEART Investigators. J Am Coll Cardiol 1991; 18(3): 647–56

36. Elezi S, Kastrati A, Neumann FJ et al. Vessel size and long-term outcome after coronary stent placement. Circulation 1998; 98(18): 1875–80

37. Kastrati A, Schomig A, Dirschinger J et al. A randomized trial comparing stenting with balloon angioplasty in small vessels in patients with symptomatic coronary artery disease. Circulation 2000; 102(21): 2593–98

38. Azar AJ, Detre K, Goldberg S et al. A meta-analysis on the clinical and angiographic outcomes of stents vs PTCA in the different coronary vessel sizes in the BENESTENT-1 and STRESS-1/2 trials. Circulation 1995; 92: I-475

39. Savage MP, Fischman DL, Rake R et al. Efficacy of coronary stenting versus balloon angioplasty in small coronary arteries. Stent Restenosis Study (STRESS) Investigators. J Am Coll Cardiol 1998; 31(2): 307–11

40. Mehilli J, Kastrati A, Dirschinger J et al. Comparison of stenting with balloon angioplasty for lesions of small coronary vessels in patients with diabetes mellitus. Am J Med 2002; 112(1): 13–18

41. Doucet S, Schalik MJ, Vrolix MC et al. Stent placement to prevent restenosis after angioplasty in small coronary arteries. Circulation 2001; 104(17): 2029–33

42. Hausleiter J, Kastrati A, Mehilli J et al. Comparative analysis of stent placement versus balloon angioplasty in small coronary arteries with long narrowings (the Intracoronary Stenting or Angioplasty for Restenosis Reduction in Small Arteries [ISAR-SMART] Trial). Am J Cardiol 2002; 89(1): 58–60

43. Holmes DR Jr, Leon MB, Moses JW et al. Analysis of 1-year clinical outcomes in the SIRIUS trial: a randomized trial of a sirolimus-eluting stent versus a standard stent in patients at high risk for coronary restenosis. Circulation 2004; 109(5): 634–40

44. Stone GW, Ellis SG, Cox DA et al. One-year clinical results with the slow-release, polymer-based, paclitaxel-eluting TAXUS stent: the TAXUS-IV trial. Circulation 2004; 109(16): 1942–47

45. Lemos PA, Arampatzis CA, Saia F et al. Treatment of very small vessels with 2.25-mm diameter sirolimus-eluting stents (from the RESEARCH registry). Am J Cardiol 2004; 93(5): 633–36

46. Saia F, Lemos PA, Arampatzis CA et al. Clinical and angiographic outcomes after overdilatation of undersized sirolimus-eluting stents with largely oversized balloons: an observational study. Catheter Cardiovasc Interv 2004; 61(4): 455–60

47. Wong SC, Baim DS, Schatz TA et al. Immediate results and late outcomes after stent implantation in saphenous vein graft lesions: the multicenter US Palmaz–Schatz stent experience. The Palmaz–Schatz Stent Study Group. J Am Coll Cardiol 1995; 26(3): 704–12

48. Brener SJ, Ellis SG, Apperson-Hansen C et al. Comparison of stenting and balloon angioplasty for narrowings in aortocoronary saphenous vein conduits in place for more than five years. Am J Cardiol 1997; 79(1): 13–18

49. Savage MP, Douglas JS, Jr., Fischman DL et al. Stent placement compared with balloon angioplasty for obstructed coronary bypass grafts. Saphenous Vein De Novo Trial Investigators. N Engl J Med 1997; 337(11): 740–47

50. Ellis SG, Guetta V, Miller D et al. Relation between lesion characteristics and risk with percutaneous intervention in the stent and glycoprotein IIb/IIIa era: an analysis of results from 10,907 lesions and proposal for new classification scheme. Circulation 1999; 100(19): 1971–76

51. Stone GW, Rogers C, Hermiller J et al. Randomized comparison of distal protection with a filter-based catheter and a balloon occlusion and aspiration system during percutaneous intervention of diseased saphenous vein aortocoronary bypass grafts. Circulation 2003; 108(5): 548–53

52. Stone GW, Cox DA, Babb J et al. Prospective, randomized evaluation of thrombectomy prior to percutaneous intervention in diseased saphenous vein grafts and thrombus-containing coronary arteries. J Am Coll Cardiol 2003; 42(11): 2007–13

53. Schachinger V, Hamm CW, Munzel T et al. A randomized trial of polytetrafluoroethylene membrane-covered stents compared with conventional stents in aortocoronary saphenous vein grafts. J Am Coll Cardiol 2003; 42(8): 1360–69

54. Ribeiro PA, Scavetta K, Oh C et al. Long-term clinical results after stent implantation in old obstructed saphenous vein grafts. Chest 2000; 118(3): 750–55

55. Kandzari DE, Goldberg S, Schwartz RS et al. Clinical and angiographic efficacy of a self-expanding nitinol stent in saphenous vein graft atherosclerotic disease: the Stent Comparative Restenosis (SCORES) Saphenous Vein Graft Registry. Am Heart J 2003; 145(5): 868–74

# 9. COMPLICATIONS RELATED TO DRUG-ELUTING STENTS

## Jose A Silva

## Introduction

Since the US Food and Drug Administration (FDA) approved drug-eluting stents (DES) for the treatment of coronary artery disease in April 2003, the use of these devices has increased exponentially. By October of 2003, more than 250 000 sirolimus-eluting stents had been implanted in the USA alone.[1]

Several prospective randomized trials have demonstrated that these devices are very effective in reducing the incidence of restenosis and are safe.[2–4] Additionally, the efficacy and safety of DES have been confirmed in clinical trials in 'real world' patients.[5]

Although the complication rates with these devices are comparable to bare metal stents (BMS), it is likely that complications will be encountered more often as their use increases. Some complications, such as subacute thrombosis, can cause significant morbidity or death. This is the reason why cardiologists and primary care physicians, who routinely follow these patients after the procedure, must be vigilant.

## Toxicity and allergy

### Systemic reactions

The drug carrier selected for the sirolimus DES (Cypher™, Cordis Johnson & Johnson, Miami, FL) is a combination of proven biostable polymers, which have been used extensively in biomedical applications and have previously been shown to be both safe and durable. The drug is mixed with the polymers, and the mixture forms a thin coat (5–10 μm thick) over the stent surface. Drug release is governed by principles of simple diffusion and results in an early burst release, followed by a secondary slower release. Because sirolimus is water insoluble (i.e. lipophilic), almost no drug is released into the bloodstream during stent advancement to the lesion site. After stent implantation, the diffusion gradient favors elution into the tissue, thereby limiting the amount of circulating sirolimus.

In the SIRIUS trial, in the subgroup of patients with long lesions or diffuse disease requiring overlapping stents ($n = 340$), no local or systemic toxicity to rapamycin was reported. On the other hand, the FDA has reported more than 70 cases of possible hypersensitivity reactions to the Cypher™ DES, consisting of pain, rash, respiratory distress, hives, itching, fever, blood pressure changes, and death. The FDA has not obtained sufficient data to establish whether these rates are different from those experienced with BMS, and therefore no specific recommendations have been made regarding this complication.[1]

## Local reactions

Concern has been raised over the possibility of the drug or polymer causing arterial wall inflammation.[6] A case of localized hypersensitivity vasculitis in response to a Cypher™ coronary stent, resulting in acute MI secondary to late acute stent thrombosis, 18 months following stent placement has been described.[7] In this report, the inflammatory cells included T-lymphocyte infiltration, with scattered B lymphocytes, and extensive eosinophilic infiltration in the intimal, media, and adventitia, particularly around the stent struts (Figures 9.1 and 9.2).

# Stent thrombosis

## Acute stent thrombosis

Intraprocedural stent thrombosis (thrombus formation during stent implantation) occurs rarely, and has been described in the setting of acute MI, in thrombus-containing lesions as well as in peri-stent dissections.[8] In a single

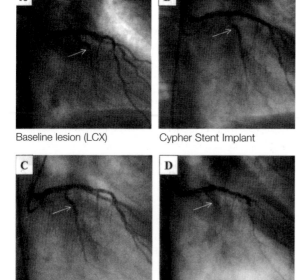

Baseline lesion (LCX)

Cypher Stent Implant

Follow-up (8 months)

Follow-up (18 months)

**Figure 9.1:** Late stent thrombosis as a consequence of the inflammatory reaction toward the Cypher™ stent. Localized hypersensitive inflammatory reaction with a Cypher™ stent. (Reproduced with permission from Virmani R, Guagliumi G, Farb A et al. Circulation 2004; 109: 701–705.)[7]

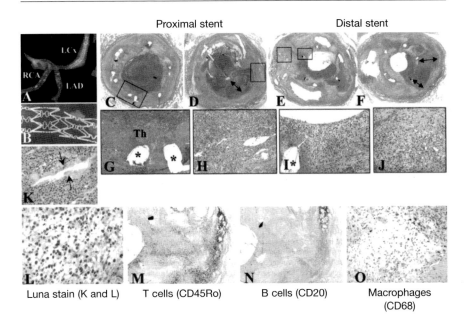

Proximal stent            Distal stent

Luna stain (K and L)    T cells (CD45Ro)    B cells (CD20)    Macrophages
(CD68)

Figure 9.2: Post mortem images of the coronary arteries, and stents. Localized hypersensitive inflammatory reaction with a Cypher™ stent. Stent malapposition is present with a space between the vessel wall and the struts (arrows) (e and f). Inflammatory cells are present (k, l, m, n, and o). (Reproduced with permission from Virmani R, Guagliumi G, Farb A et al. Circulation 2004; 109: 701–705.)[7]

center report, intraprocedural stent thrombosis occurred in five (0.7%) of 670 patients treated with Cypher™ stents.[9] None of these patients had been treated with platelet GP IIb/IIIa inhibitors during the procedure, and all patients showed stent under-expansion with intravascular ultrasound (IVUS). However, using logistic regression analysis, only total stent length per vessel was associated with the occurrence of intraprocedural stent thrombosis. The consequences were dire in four of the five patients who developed this complication: three patients had an acute MI (one patient Q-wave MI), and one patient died during emergent surgical revascularization.

## Subacute stent thrombosis

Subacute stent thrombosis is defined as the occurrence of stent thrombosis within the first 30 days after stent implantation. This has become a relatively rare complication (0.5 to 2%) with the routine use of high-pressure balloon inflation for stent deployment and pretreatment with a thienopyridine antiplatelet agent in combination with aspirin.[10] This complication has the potential to be catastrophic, with a mortality rate from 5 to 20%, an MI rate of 43 to 100%, and the need for emergent bypass surgery in up to 50%.[11]

In October 2003, the FDA received more than 290 reports (over 260 in the USA and over 25 outside the USA) of subacute stent thrombosis associated with Cypher™ stent implantation. More than 60 cases were associated with the patient's death, and the rest were associated with MI requiring percutaneous or surgical intervention. At this time, more than 450 000 stents had been deployed worldwide. After review of the available data, the FDA concluded that the rate of subacute stent thrombosis was not different from that experienced with BMS.[1]

Two recent reports have documented that subacute stent thrombosis with the Cypher™ stent is not higher than with BMS. In a single center experience of 652 Cypher™ stents, deployed from April 2003 through October 2003, seven patients (1.1%; range 2–13 days) developed subacute stent thrombosis, and one patient developed late stent thrombosis.[12] Of the seven patients with subacute stent thrombosis, five patients had a MI, and one patient died. The only differences between patients with and without subacute stent thrombosis were smaller final balloon diameters (2.75 versus 3.0 mm; $P = 0.04$), and discontinuation of antiplatelet therapy (57 versus 1.7%; $P < 0.001$). In a second report of 510 consecutive patients treated with Cypher™ stents, two patients (0.4%) developed subacute stent thrombosis 6 hours and 11 days after the procedure.[13] Both cases occurred in diabetic women with complex coronary lesions, and IVUS had demonstrated inadequate stent expansion and an uncovered distal dissection. These data confirm that the use of DES deployed to ensure optimal stent expansion and with the appropriate antiplatelet regimen are not associated with an increased incidence of subacute stent thrombosis. A case of subacute stent thrombosis is shown in Figure 9.3.

## Late stent thrombosis

Late stent thrombosis is defined as acute thrombotic occlusion occurring later than 30 days after stent implantation. Late stent thrombosis is a well-recognized complication after coronary brachytherapy, due to impaired endothelialization.[14] A recent study of 168 stented native coronary arteries identified 13 patients with late stent thrombosis (7.7%).[15] The pathologic mechanisms associated with this complication were:

- stenting across the ostia of major arterial branches
- plaque disruption within 2 mm of the stent margin
- exposure to radiation therapy
- stenting of markedly necrotic, lipid-rich plaques, with extensive plaque prolapse
- diffuse in-stent restentosis (ISR).

The use of DES has also been identified as a cause of late stent thrombosis, presumably due to impaired or delayed endothelialization as it

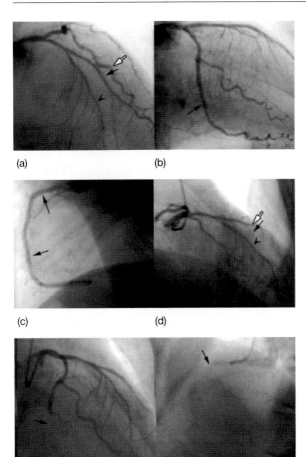

(a)          (b)

(c)          (d)

(e)          (f)

Figure 9.3: An angiogram of a 91-year-old patient with multivessel DES placement. (a) Left anterior descending (LAD) (black arrow), diagonal branch (white arrow), and a septal perforator (arrowhead). (b) Circumflex (LCx) stent location (black arrow). (c) Location of the stent in the right coronary artery (RCA). Eight days later, the patient presented with cardiogenic shock – an angiogram revealed stent thrombosis of all the stents. (d) LAD (black arrow) occlusion. (e) LCX occlusion. (f) RCA stent closure.

occurs with brachytherapy, or due to the development of hypersensitivity vasculitis.[7,16] However, the data show that this complication occurs at the same frequency as with BMS. Pooled data from RAVEL, SIRIUS, E-SIRIUS, and C-SIRIUS, reported an incidence of late stent thrombosis of 0.1% (0.5% for the control arm).[3] Likewise, in the previously mentioned US and European single-center registries of more than 1100 patients, there was only one case of late stent thrombosis reported.[13]

These data demonstrate the similarity for what occurs with BMS, and that late stent thrombosis is a rare occurrence after the use of DES. However, because of the delayed endothelialization with the use of DES, it is recommended that aspirin in combination with clopidogrel or ticlopidine be used for at least six months. A case of late stent thrombosis secondary to a local inflammatory reaction is shown in Figure 9.1b.

## Under-expansion and incomplete stent apposition

### Stent under-expansion

Incomplete stent expansion and poor apposition against the vessel wall is a strong predictor for ISR and stent thrombosis after the deployment of BMS.[17] With appropriate sizing, using the appropriate balloon-to-vessel ratio and the use of high-pressure balloon inflation, it was demonstrated that adequate stent expansion could be accomplished in the majority of the cases, and routine use of IVUS was not necessary.[18]

Stent under-expansion appears to be a strong predictor of ISR after the deployment of sirolimus-eluting stents. An IVUS subanalysis from SIRIUS of 126 patients found that a minimum stent area of less than 5 mm$^2$ was the threshold for target lesion revascularization (TLR) eight months after treatment of de-novo lesions.[18] Stent under-expansion is a strong predictor for recurrent ISR, after treatment of the first ISR with sirolimus-eluting stents.[19] These data suggest that optimal stent expansion of DES is as important to reduce the restenosis rate as it is for BMS.

### Incomplete stent apposition

Incomplete stent apposition is a separation of the stent struts from the intimal surface of the arterial wall that was not present after stent implantation. It usually occurs as a result of positive remodeling without an increase in plaque mass. Studies with IVUS have shown an increased radius of the external elastic membrane at site of the malapposed stent.[20] Late stent malapposition occurs in 4 to 5% of BMS, and appears to be more frequent with DES.[21] In the RAVEL trial as well as in the SIRIUS trial, late stent malapposition was found to be significantly higher in the Cypher™ stent group compared to the control BMS group (Figure 9.4).[22,23]

At one-year follow-up of the RAVEL incomplete stent expansion patients, there were no adverse events found in this group. The vessel dimensions surrounding the incomplete stent apposition area did not change over time, except for one patient who developed an aneurysm.[24]

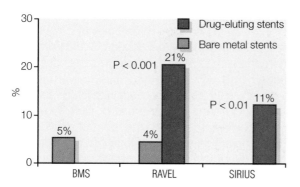

**Figure 9.4:** Late stent incomplete apposition, in bare metal stents (BMS)[21] and in two prospective randomized trials comparing sirolimus-eluting stents and BMS.[22,23]

## Coronary aneurysm formation

Although the rate of incomplete stent apposition is increased in vessels treated with sirolimus-eluting stents compared to BMS, the data have failed to show that aneurysm formation is higher after deployment of sirolimus-eluting stents. Only one coronary aneurysm was observed in the group of 13 RAVEL patients with incomplete stent apposition after one-year of follow-up.[24] This patient was treated successfully with a covered stent, and had an uneventful clinical outcome (Figures 9.5 and 9.6).

## Conclusion

Drug-eluting stents have been welcomed worldwide, and at present more than half a million devices have been implanted successfully. Although no systemic or local adverse reactions to rapamycin or paclitaxel have been reported, a few patients have developed a systemic hypersensitivity reaction

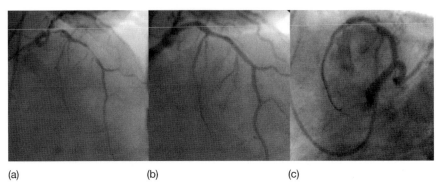

(a)          (b)          (c)

Figure 9.5: (a) Baseline angiogram showing tight ostial and mid LAD stenoses. (b) After successful placement of two sirolimus-eluting stents in the proximal and mid portions of the LAD. (c) Left anterior descending caudal view after stent placement.

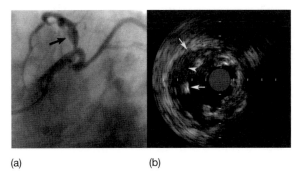

Figure 9.6: (a) Proximal LAD aneurysm three months after stent placement. (b) IVUS image showing non-apposition of the stent struts (upper and lower arrows, respectively) with the vessel wall and the aneurysm (arrowhead).

(a)          (b)

101

whose cause remains to be determined. One case of allergic vasculitis of the arterial wall has been reported which had a fatal outcome after the patient developed late stent thrombosis. Late incomplete stent apposition appears to be more frequent in vessels treated with sirolimus-eluting stents. However, this complication has not increased cardiovascular events, or enhanced the likelihood of aneurysm formation. Finally, several studies have now confirmed that the potentially lethal complication of subacute or late stent thrombosis is not increased with the use of DES with optimal stent deployment and an antiplatelet regimen of clopidogrel or ticlopidine in combination with aspirin for at least six months.

# References

1. FDA advises physicians of adverse events associated with the Cordis Cypher coronary stents. US Food and Drug Administration Public Health Web Notification. 29 October 2003; T03–T71; 2003 (accessed at http://www.fda.gov/cdrh/safety/cypher3.html#footnote)

2. Morice MC, Serruys PW, Sousa JE et al. A randomized comparison of a sirolimus-eluting stent with a standard stent for coronary revascularization. N Engl J Med 2002; 346(23): 1773–80

3. Moses JW, Leon MB, Popma JJ et al. Sirolimus-eluting stents versus standard stents in patients with stenosis in a native coronary artery. N Engl J Med 2003; 349(14): 1315–23

4. Park SJ, Shim WH, Ho DS et al. A paclitaxel-eluting stent for the prevention of coronary restenosis. N Engl J Med 2003; 348(16): 1537–45

5. Lemos PA, Hoye A, Goedhart D et al. Clinical, angiographic, and procedural predictors of angiographic restenosis after sirolimus-eluting stent implantation in complex patients: an evaluation from the Rapamycin-Eluting Stent Evaluated At Rotterdam Cardiology Hospital (RESEARCH) study. Circulation 2004; 109(11): 1366–70

6. Van der Giessen WJ, Lincoff AM, Schwartz RS et al. Marked inflammatory sequelae to implantation of biodegradable and nonbiodegradable polymers in porcine coronary arteries. Circulation 1996; 94(7): 1690–97

7. Virmani R, Guagliumi G, Farb A et al. Localized hypersensitivity and late coronary thrombosis secondary to a sirolimus-eluting stent: should we be cautious? Circulation 2004; 109(6): 701–705

8. Schuhlen H, Kastrati A, Dirschinger J et al. Intracoronary stenting and risk for major adverse cardiac events during the first month. Circulation 1998; 98(2): 104–11

9. Chieffo A, Bonizzoni E, Orlic D et al. Intraprocedural stent thrombosis during implantation of sirolimus-eluting stents. Circulation 2004; 109(22): 2732–36

10. Colombo A, Hall P, Nakamura S et al. Intracoronary stenting without anticoagulation accomplished with intravascular ultrasound guidance. Circulation 1995; 91(6): 1676–88

11. Hasdai D, Garratt KN, Holmes DR Jr et al. Coronary angioplasty and intracoronary thrombolysis are of limited efficacy in resolving early intracoronary stent thrombosis. J Am Coll Cardiol 1996; 28(2): 361–67

12. Jeremias A, Sylvia B, Bridges J et al. Stent thrombosis after successful sirolimus-eluting stent implantation. Circulation 2004; 109(16): 1930–32

13. Regar E, Lemos PA, Saia F et al. Incidence of thrombotic stent occlusion during the first three months after sirolimus-eluting stent implantation in 500 consecutive patients. Am J Cardiol 2004; 93(10): 1271–75

14. Costa MA, Sabat M, van der Giessen WJ et al. Late coronary occlusion after intracoronary brachytherapy. Circulation 1999; 100(8): 789–92

15. Farb A, Burke AP, Kolodgie FD et al. Pathological mechanisms of fatal late coronary stent thrombosis in humans. Circulation 2003; 108(14): 1701–706

16. Liistro F, Colombo A. Late acute thrombosis after paclitaxel-eluting stent implantation. Heart 2001; 86(3): 262–64

17. Sick P, Huttl T, Niebauer J et al. Influence of residual stenosis after percutaneous coronary intervention with stent implantation on development of restenosis and stent thrombosis. Am J Cardiol 2003; 91(2): 148–53

18. Sonoda S, Morino Y, Ako J et al. An optimal diagnostic threshold of minimum stent area to predict long-term stent patency following sirolimus-eluting stent implantation: serial intravascular ultrasound analysis from SIRIUS trial. J Am Coll Cardiol 2003; 41: 80A

19. Fujii K, Mintz GS, Kobayashi Y et al. Contribution of stent underexpansion to recurrence after sirolimus-eluting stent implantation for in-stent restenosis. Circulation 2004; 109(9): 1085–88

20. Mintz GS, Shah VM, Weissman NJ. Regional remodeling as the cause of late stent malapposition. Circulation 2003; 107(21): 2660–63

21. Shah VM, Mintz GS, Apple S et al. Background incidence of late malapposition after bare-metal stent implantation. Circulation 2002; 106(14): 1753–55

22. Serruys PW, Degertekin M, Tanabe K et al. Intravascular ultrasound findings in the multicenter, randomized, double-blind RAVEL (RAndomized study with the sirolimus-eluting VElocity balloon-expandable stent in the treatment of patients with de novo native coronary artery Lesions) trial. Circulation 2002; 106(7): 798–803

23. Ako J, Morino Y, Honda Y et al. Late incomplete stent apposition following sirolimus-eluting stent: serial quantitative intravascular ultrasound analysis from the SIRIUS trial. J Am Coll Cardiol 2003; 41: 33A

24. Degertekin M, Serruys PW, Tanabe K et al. Long-term follow-up of incomplete stent apposition in patients who received sirolimus-eluting stent for de novo coronary lesions: an intravascular ultrasound analysis. Circulation 2003; 108(22): 2747–50

# PART IV

# OPTIMAL PATIENT MANAGEMENT AND SELECTION FOR DRUG-ELUTING STENTS

# 10. PATIENT SELECTION CRITERIA FOR DRUG-ELUTING STENTS

Ali Morshedi-Meibodi and J Stephen Jenkins

## Introduction

Since the introduction of coronary angioplasty by Andrea Gruntzig in 1977, the long-term durability of this procedure has been limited by recurrent narrowing within the stent: restenosis. The emergence of coronary stents proved superior to balloon angioplasty alone for long-term vessel patency.[1,2] The invention of drug-eluting stents (DES) was another leap forward in further reducing the restenosis rate. First-in-man studies demonstrated striking reductions in clinical restenosis.[3] The first major clinical trial examining the durable patency of DES was the Randomized Study with the Sirolimus-Eluting Bx Velocity Balloon-ExpandabLe stent (RAVEL).[4] This trial was followed by the pivotal US Food and Drug Administration (FDA) approval trial SIRollmUS (SIRIUS)-coated stent in the treatment of patients with de-novo coronary artery lesions, that resulted in approval of DES by the FDA in October 2002.[5]

The pivotal FDA approval trials for DES were conducted on single lesions in native coronary arteries. Patient selection was carefully restricted by lesion characteristics and clinical presentation. The RAVEL trial selection criteria included a clinical diagnosis of stable angina, unstable angina, or silent ischemia in native vessels with single lesions, with a diameter of 2.5–3.5 mm; stenoses of 51% to 99% were included. Subjects with evolving myocardial infarction (MI), left main coronary artery disease, ostial lesions, heavily calcified lesions, and thrombus-containing lesions were excluded. The results of the RAVEL trial were unprecedented with a reduction in restenosis to zero compared to 26.6% (P < 0.001) in the bare metal stent (BMS) group.[4]

The inclusion criteria for the FDA pivotal trial for the paclitaxel-coated stent, TAXUS IV, were similar to RAVEL; however, lesion characteristics were extended to include larger diameters (2.5–3.75 mm) and longer lesions (10–28 mm).[6] In this study the rate of angiographic restenosis was 26.6% in the BMS control group and 7.9% in the DES group (P < 0.001). One-year follow-up revealed a reduction of target lesion revascularization (TLR) from 11.3% in the BMS group to 3% in the DES group (P < 0.001).

After DES became available for clinical use in Europe, they were implanted in a much broader range of clinical scenarios than those originally represented by the pivotal trial patients. The Rapamycin-Eluting Stent

Evaluated At Rotterdam Cardiology Hospital (RESEARCH) study evaluated the use of sirolimus-eluting stent (SES) implantation in this broader group of lesions.[7] In this registry, DES were placed in high-risk lesions subsets, i.e. bifurcations, long lesions, chronic total occlusions, small vessels, left main coronary arteries, and acute MI. In this high-risk registry, the six-month restenosis rate (7.9%) was lower than that expected for historic controls in complex lesions (43% based on meta-analysis of studies with BMS).[8,9]

Multivariate analysis of this registry revealed that independent predictors of restenosis were ostial lesions, left anterior descending artery location, presence of diabetes mellitus, stent length, and reference diameter (Table 10.1). In comparison to low-risk lesions, treatment of high-risk lesions with DES was associated with higher absolute risk reduction (Figure 10.1). By highlighting the efficacy of DES in high-risk lesions, the RESEARCH registry set the stage for further investigation in lesions at risk for restenosis.

## Drug-eluting stents for in-stent restenosis

Several studies have examined the use of DES as a treatment for in-stent restenosis (ISR). One study in 16 patients evaluated the use of DES for treatment of severe recurrent ISR in native coronary arteries with objective evidence of ischemia.[10] Late lumen loss within the stent at four months was lower than the historical control with BMS (0.21 mm vs 1.36 mm) or rotational atherectomy followed by beta radiation (0.37 mm). During the nine-month follow-up, three of 16 patients had major adverse cardiac events (MACE).

Sousa et al. found similar results with the use of sirolimus DES for the treatment of ISR.[11] In this study, late lumen loss was 0.36 mm at 12-month follow-up. The restenosis rate was only 4% with no deaths, no stent thromboses, and no repeat revascularizations. TAXUS III examined the use of paclitaxel-eluting stents for the treatment of ISR.[12] Late lumen loss was decreased to 0.54 mm at six-month follow-up. Restenosis occurred in the gap

| Table 10.1. Multivariate odds ratio for restenosis in the RESEARCH registry | |
|---|---|
| *High-risk lesions* | *Odds ratio for restenosis* |
| Ostial location | 4.84 |
| Restenosis | 4.16 |
| Diabetes mellitus | 2.63 |
| Total stent length* | 1.42 |
| Reference diameter[†] | 0.46 |
| LAD | 0.3 |

*Per 10 mm increase; [†]Per 1.0 mm decrease.

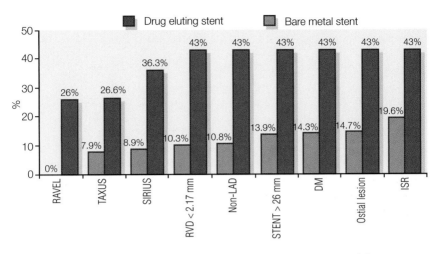

Figure 10.1: Comparison of restenosis with DES among various risk groups.[4–9]

between paclitaxel-eluting stents in four (16%) patients. Analysis of the stented area directly exposed to paclitaxel revealed that late lumen loss was actually lower (0.47 mm) and the restenosis rate was only 4.5%. Lesions treated with a single stent demonstrated a late lumen loss of 0.36 mm, similar to the late loss in de-novo lesions treated with paclitaxel-eluting stents in TAXUS I.[13] Subjects receiving two stents had a higher rate of restenosis. The rate of MACE was 29% during the six-month follow-up. An intravascular ultrasound (IVUS) substudy confirmed the lack of any positive or negative remodeling. Table 10.2 compares the different modalities for treatment of ISR.[14,15] While these trials revealed a decrease in late lumen loss with DES, they were inconsistent with regard to a decrease in the rate of clinical end-points.

| Table 10.2. Comparison of different modalities for the treatment of in-stent restenosis | | | |
|---|---|---|---|
| Modalities | Lumen loss (mm) | Restenosis (%) | Duration of follow-up (months) |
| PTCA[14] | 1.07 | 45.2 | 11 |
| Bare metal stent[14] | 1.36 | 41.4 | 11 |
| Rotational atherectomy[14] | 1.30 | 35.9 | 11 |
| Cutting balloon[14] | 0.63 | 20 | 11 |
| Atherectomy/radiation[15] | 0.37 | 10 | 10 |
| TAXUS III[12] | 0.56 | 16 | 6 |
| DES[11] | 0.36 | 4 | 12 |
| DES[10] | 0.21 | 6.7 | 4 |

## Drug-eluting stents in acute coronary syndromes

The RESEARCH registry reported results of sirolimus DES in patients with acute coronary syndromes (ACS).[16] There was a lower rate of MACE (death, MI, target vessel revascularization) at 300 days in the DES group compared to the BMS group (9.4% vs 17%); P = 0.02). The lower MACE rate was due in large part to a decrease in target vessel revascularization (TVR). Although increased stent thrombosis is a theoretical concern in ACS, none of the subjects in the DES group had stent thrombosis compared to 1.6% in the control group (P = 0.1).

## Drug-eluting stents in bifurcation lesions

Bifurcation lesions have been historically associated with a higher rate of restenosis and adverse events. The use of DES in bifurcation stenting has been studied by Colombo and colleagues who compared historical controls to simultaneous stenting of the main branch and stenting the side-branch (stent/stent) compared to stenting of the main branch and balloon angioplasty of the side-branch (stent/balloon).[17] Using DES, the restenosis rate was 28% in the stent/stent group compared to 18.7% in the stent/balloon group (P = 0.53). This restenosis rate is lower than for historic controls with a rate of 61.6% in the stent/stent and 48.1% in stent/balloon treatment of bifurcating lesions.[18] With DES, restenosis of the side-branch was higher in the stented group than in the balloon angioplasty group. The lower rate of restenosis in the main branch in the stent/stent group was offset by a higher rate of target vessel failure (TVF) and stent thrombosis. Subjects who were stented only in the main branch had a lower rate of TVF compared to the stent/stent group (13.6% vs 19%). These results may be due to patient selection with subjects with isolated main branch stenting having more favorable lesion morphology.

## Drug-eluting stents in small vessels

Small vessel diameter is a risk factor for restenosis. In the RESEARCH registry, reference vessel diameter (RVD) was an independent predictor of restenosis.[7] Every millimeter increase in RVD was associated with a 54% reduction in risk of restenosis. In the RAVEL study, the use of DES was compared across three strata: stratum I – RVD < 2.36 mm; stratum II – RVD 2.36–2.84 mm; stratum III – RVD > 2.84 mm.[19] While the use of BMS was associated with restenosis rates of 35%, 26%, and 20% in strata I, II, and III, respectively, this rate remained zero in all the DES groups during six-month follow-up. Figure 10.2 compares the late lumen loss across the strata. In the RESEARCH registry, in-segment restenosis after the use of DES was 10.3% for vessels with RVD < 2.17 mm. Patient inclusion in this registry was closer to the 'real life' situation.[7]

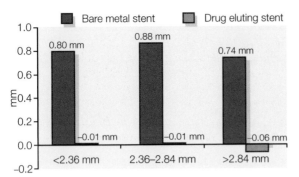

Figure 10.2: Comparison of late lumen loss across three strata.[19]

# Drug-eluting stents in diabetics with multivessel disease

Diabetes is a major risk factor for ISR. Traditionally patients with diabetes and multivessel coronary disease have been referred for coronary bypass surgery. The Future REvascularization Evaluation in Diabetes Optimal Management (FREEDOM) trial, sponsored by the National Institute of Health, will compare bypass surgery to the use of DES in diabetic patients with multivessel disease.[20]

# Conclusion

Patients should be selected for DES in a methodical fashion based upon the risk of restenosis. Predictors of restenosis can be classified in three categories: clinical; lesion; and procedural factors. Patient selection begins by examining the clinical predictors of restenosis (Box 10.1). Diagnostic coronary angiography reveals lesion characteristics that increase the propensity for restenosis to occur. Patients at increased risk of restenosis should be considered candidates for a DES unless procedural factors dictate otherwise. In the absence of clinical predictors of restenosis or high-risk lesion characteristics, BMS may be preferred.

**Box 10.1 Predictors of restenosis**

- Clinical predictors:
  - diabetes mellitus
  - prior restenosis
- Lesion characteristics:
  - lesion length
  - reference vessel diameter
  - ostial lesion location
  - saphenous vein graft lesions
  - bifurcation lesions
  - non-left anterior descending (LAD) coronary artery lesions
  - minimal luminal diameter post-stenting
- Procedural predictors:
  - number of stents
  - length of stent

# References

1. Fischman DL, Leon MB, Baim DS et al. A randomized comparison of coronary-stent placement and balloon angioplasty in the treatment of coronary artery disease. Stent Restenosis Study Investigators. N Engl J Med 1994; 331(8): 496–501

2. Serruys PW, de Jaegere P, Kiemeneij F et al. A comparison of balloon-expandable stent implantation with balloon angioplasty in patients with coronary artery disease. Benestent Study Group. N Engl J Med 1994; 331(8): 489–95

3. Sousa JE, Costa MA, Abizaid AC et al. Sustained suppression of neointimal proliferation by sirolimus-eluting stents: one-year angiographic and intravascular ultrasound follow-up. Circulation 2001; 104(17): 2007–11

4. Morice MC, Serruys PW, Sousa JE et al. A randomized comparison of a sirolimus-eluting stent with a standard stent for coronary revascularization. N Engl J Med 2002; 346(23): 1773–80

5. Moses JW, Leon MB, Popma JJ et al. Sirolimus-eluting stents versus standard stents in patients with stenosis in a native coronary artery. N Engl J Med 2003; 349(14): 1315–23

6. Stone GW, Ellis SG, Cox DA et al. A polymer-based, paclitaxel-eluting stent in patients with coronary artery disease. N Engl J Med 2004; 350(3): 221–31

7. Lemos PA, Hoye A, Goedhart D et al. Clinical, angiographic, and procedural predictors of angiographic restenosis after sirolimus-eluting stent implantation in complex patients: an evaluation from the Rapamycin-Eluting Stent Evaluated At Rotterdam Cardiology Hospital (RESEARCH) study. Circulation 2004; 109(11): 1366–70

8. Ho KKL, Senerchia C, Rodriguez O et al. Predictors of angiographic restenosis after stenting: pooled analysis of 1197 patient with protocol-mandated angiographic follow-up from 5 randomized stent trials (abstract). Circulation 1998; 98 (Suppl I): I-362

9. Mercado N, Boersma E, Wijns W et al. Clinical and quantitative coronary angiographic predictors of coronary restenosis: a comparative analysis from the balloon-to-stent era. J Am Coll Cardiol 2001; 38(3): 645–52

10. Degertekin M, Regar E, Tanabe K et al. Sirolimus-eluting stent for treatment of complex in-stent restenosis: the first clinical experience. J Am Coll Cardiol 2003; 41(2): 184–89

11. Sousa JE, Costa MA, Abizaid A et al. Sirolimus-eluting stent for the treatment of in-stent restenosis: a quantitative coronary angiography and three-dimensional intravascular ultrasound study. Circulation 2003; 107(1): 24–27

12. Tanabe K, Serruys PW, Grube E et al. TAXUS III Trial: in-stent restenosis treated with stent-based delivery of paclitaxel incorporated in a slow-release polymer formulation. Circulation 2003; 107(4): 559–64

13. Grube E, Silber S, Hauptmann KE et al. TAXUS I: six- and twelve-month results from a randomized, double-blind trial on a slow-release paclitaxel-eluting stent for de novo coronary lesions. Circulation 2003; 107(1): 38–42

14. Adamian M, Colombo A, Briguori C et al. Cutting balloon angioplasty for the treatment of in-stent restenosis: a matched comparison with rotational atherectomy, additional stent implantation and balloon angioplasty. J Am Coll Cardiol 2001; 38(3): 672–79

15. Park SW, Hong MK, Moon DH et al. Treatment of diffuse in-stent restenosis with rotational atherectomy followed by radiation therapy with a rhenium-188 mercaptoacetyltriglycine-filled balloon. J Am Coll Cardiol 2001; 38(3): 631–37

16. Lemos PA, Saia F, Hofma SH et al. Short- and long-term clinical benefit of sirolimus-eluting stents compared to conventional bare stents for patients with acute myocardial infarction. J Am Coll Cardiol 2004; 43(4): 704–708

17. Colombo A, Moses JW, Morice MC et al. Randomized study to evaluate sirolimus-eluting stents implanted at coronary bifurcation lesions. Circulation 2004; 109(10): 1244–49

18. Yamashita T, Nishida T, Adamian MG et al. Bifurcation lesions: two stents versus one stent – immediate and follow-up results. J Am Coll Cardiol 2000; 35(5): 1145–51

19. Regar E, Serruys PW, Bode C et al. Angiographic findings of the multicenter Randomized Study With the Sirolimus-Eluting Bx Velocity Balloon-Expandable Stent (RAVEL): sirolimus-eluting stents inhibit restenosis irrespective of the vessel size. Circulation 2002; 106(15): 1949–56

20. Teirstein PS. A chicken in every pot and a drug-eluting stent in every lesion. Circulation 2004; 109(16): 1906–10

# 11. OPTIMAL ANTIPLATELET AND ANTICOAGULATION THERAPY FOR DRUG-ELUTING STENTS

Mahesh S Mulumudi and Tyrone J Collins

## Introduction

The major limitations of percutaneous transluminal coronary angioplasty (PTCA) are acute vessel closure and restenosis. The advent of intracoronary stents resulted in a significant reduction in these complications.[1,2] Improvements in the stent design, deployment techniques, and post-interventional antithrombotic therapy reduced the incidence of acute and subacute stent thrombosis from 20% to 1.3%.[3,4] Drug-eluting stents (DES) emerged as a solution to restenosis. They dramatically reduced the incidence of restenosis but raised the question of whether there is an increase in the incidence of stent thrombosis with these newer stents. In this chapter we will review the available data on the occurrence of stent thrombosis with DES and optimal antithrombotic regimens to prevent it.

## Pathophysiology

Stents are inherently thrombogenic.[5,6] They markedly enhance the platelet activation and coagulation cascade that occurs at the injured plaque in the vessel. The exposure of the procoagulant subendothelial structures that occur after angioplasty causes contact activation of the kinin-generation system. Subsequent tissue factor presentation causes thrombin generation and platelet activation. Platelet activation peaks on the second day after coronary stenting.[7] Activated platelets bind with plasma fibrinogen leading to platelet aggregation and thrombus generation through interplatelet bridging.[8]

## Stent thrombosis with drug-eluting stents

With the widespread use of DES, questions regarding the incidence of stent thrombosis emerged. An initial hint of stent thrombosis with DES was seen in ASPECT (the ASian Paclitaxel-Eluting stent Clinical Trial), which used a paclitaxel-covered stent.[9] All four cases of stent thrombosis occurred in the group receiving aspirin and cilostazol but not in patients receiving aspirin plus clopidogrel/ticlopidine. This probably reflected inadequate antiplatelet therapy rather than a primary problem with the drug-coated stents.

Stent thrombosis did not occur at an increased rate compared to bare metal stents (BMS) in trials using DES and double antiplatelet therapy with aspirin plus ticolopidine/clopidogrel. In the SIRIUS (Sirolimus-Coated Bx VELOCITY Balloon-Expandable Stent) trial there was no difference in the occurrence of stent thrombosis between the sirolimus and the control groups.[10] In this trial acute (<24 hours) stent thrombosis did not occur in either the sirolimus or BMS groups. Subacute (1–30 days) stent thrombosis occurred in one patient (1/533; 0.2%) in the sirolimus group and in one patient (1/525; 0.2%) in the control group. Late (31–270 days) stent thrombosis happened in one patient (1/533; 0.2%) in the sirolimus group and in one patient (1/525; 0.2%) in the control group. The total number of patients who developed stent thrombosis was two (0.4%) and four (0.8%) in the sirolimus-eluting stent (SES) and control BMS groups, respectively.

Examining all the sirolimus stent trials – Randomized Study With the Sirolimus-Eluting Bx VELOCITY Balloon-Expandable Stent (RAVEL), SIRIUS, E-SIRIUS, and C-SIRIUS[10–12] – a total of 878 patients were randomized to the DES arm and 870 to the BMS arm. The overall incidence of stent thrombosis was identical (0.6%) in both the sirolimus and control groups. This compares to the occurrence of stent thrombosis with BMS, a 0.8% incidence in the ISAR (Intracoronary Stenting and Antithrombotic Regimen)[13] and 0.6% incidence in the STARS (Stent Anticoagulation Regimen Study)[14] trials.

The incidence of stent thrombosis with sirolimus-coated stents in the real world registries in both the USA and abroad is below 1.5% (Figure 11.1). A total of 109 223 patients received a SES in these registries. In the TAXUS trial 662 patients received a paclitaxel-eluting stent and 652 patients received a BMS.[15] The incidence of stent thrombosis is very similar to that seen with the SES. The incidence was 0.6% (4/662) in the paclitaxel group compared to 0.8% (5/652) in the BMS group (Figure 11.2).

The incidence of stent thrombosis with both the sirolimus and paclitaxel stents is less than 1%, comparable to the incidence with BMS. In the DES trials established antithrombotic regimens were utilized. With the exception of the duration of the double antiplatelet therapy, the standard antiplatelet regimens can be safely applied to the DES implantation.

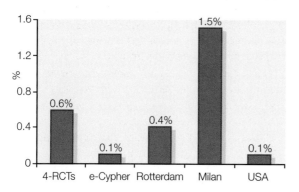

**Figure 11.1:** Sirolimus drug-eluting stent thrombosis rate in multiple trials (total of 109 223 patients).

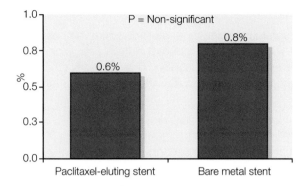

**Figure 11.2:** The incidence of stent thrombosis in the TAXUS trial.[15]

## Antithrombotic therapies

### Aspirin

Aspirin inactivates prostaglandin synthase, the first step in the conversion of arachidonic acid to thromboxane $A_2$, resulting in inhibition of prostaglandin synthesis. Antiplatelet actions of aspirin are due to the inhibition of prostaglandin synthesis. Thromboxane $A_2$ is just one of over 90 agonists that can stimulate platelet aggregation.

Aspirin is rapidly absorbed from the stomach and upper small intestine, and peak plasma levels occur in 30 to 40 minutes after ingestion. With the enteric-coated preparations it may take up to three to four hours to achieve peak plasma levels. Aspirin's plasma half-life is approximately 15–20 minutes. In spite of its rapid clearance from the circulation, the antiplatelet effect of aspirin on each platelet is permanent for the lifespan of the affected platelet; 10% of circulating platelets are replaced every 24 hours. Therefore only 50% of platelets remain inhibited at about five days after an initial loading dose of aspirin. Low-dose aspirin regimens (<160 mg/day) are equally effective as the regimens using 160 to 325 mg/day.[16,17] There is no evidence to support the use of aspirin in doses less than 75 mg/day.

Several clinical trials have demonstrated the undisputed benefits of aspirin in coronary artery disease, unstable angina, myocardial infarction (MI), and coronary angioplasty;[17] the use of aspirin during coronary angioplasty is now routine. Aspirin pretreatment reduced the incidence of angiographically detected thrombi at 30 minutes after angioplasty from 10.7% to 1.8%.[19] However, aspirin as a monotherapy for platelet inhibition after stent implantation is inadequate. This was clearly shown in the Stent Anticoagulation Regimen Study (STARS).[14] In STARS, out of a total of 1653 patients, 557 were randomized to receive aspirin alone, 546 to receive aspirin plus ticlopidine, and 550 to receive anticoagulation with warfarin plus aspirin. Major adverse cardiac events (MACE), predominantly subacute stent thrombosis, were six times higher in patients receiving aspirin alone compared to those receiving aspirin plus ticlopidine.

## Thienopyridines

The thienopyridines, clopidogrel and ticlopidine, are adenosine diphosphate (ADP) receptor antagonists. They block ADP-induced platelet activation. Their effect on platelet inhibition is synergistic with aspirin. The necessity of double platelet therapy with a thienopyridine and aspirin after stent implantation is well documented.[13,14,20,21]

### Ticlopidine

Ticlopidine is metabolised to an active compound in the liver. Being a prodrug, its onset of action is delayed, reaching a plateau by the end of the first week. In optimally deployed stents, short-term heparin plus antiplatelet therapy with ticlopidine and aspirin appear adequate to prevent stent thrombosis. The first randomized trial to compare ticlopidine plus aspirin with anticoagulation with warfarin and aspirin was the ISAR trial.[13] In this trial 517 patients were randomized to either receive ticlopidine plus aspirin or anticoagulation with warfarin plus aspirin. The stent thrombosis rate was 0.8% in the ticlopidine plus aspirin arm. The primary end-point of cardiac death, heart attack, emergent aortocoronary bypass surgery, or repeat angioplasty was seen in 1.6% of the patients with antiplatelet therapy and in 6.2% of those receiving anticoagulation. In the STARS, ticlopidine plus aspirin was superior to both the aspirin alone and warfarin plus aspirin.[14] In this study the ticlopidine plus aspirin arm had a stent thrombosis rate of 0.5%.

In both the ISAR and STARS trials Palmaz–Schatz™ (Cordis, Miami, FL) stents were used. In the FANTASTIC (Full ANTicoagulation versus Aspirin and TIClipidine) trial 485 patients were randomized to receive ticlopidine plus aspirin or warfarin anticoagulation after Wiktor™ (Medtronic, Minneapolis, MN) stent (coil design) placement.[20] The Wiktor™ stent is made of tantalum and the Palmaz–Schatz is made of stainless steel. It is apparent from these data that ticlopidine plus aspirin therapy was superior to warfarin anticoagulation (Figure 11.3). It is also apparent that the benefits of double antiplatelet therapy are not limited to a particular stent design or material. In addition, the superiority of antiplatelet therapy over anticoagulation in high-risk patients (stents implanted for abrupt closure after balloon angioplasty, suboptimal stent implantation, lesions longer than 45 mm, and largest balloon used was less than 2.5 mm) was demonstrated in the Multicenter Aspirin and Ticlopidine Trial after Intracoronary Stenting (MATTIS) trial.[21]

Ticlopidine-induced neutropenia occurs in 2.4% of the patients and usually occurs within the first three months. It can be fatal and requires prompt discontinuation of the drug. A more serious complication is thrombotic thrombocytopenic purpura-hemolytic uremic syndrome. It occurs in 1/1600 to 1/4800 cases. All cases occur within 12 weeks and 75% between 3 to 12 weeks. Treatment includes discontinuation of the drug and plasmapheresis. Because of the seriousness of the complications it is imperative that blood

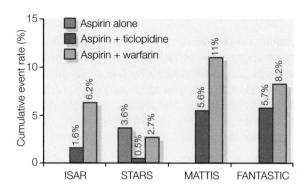

Figure 11.3: It is apparent from these data that ticlopidine plus aspirin therapy was superior to warfarin anticoagulation for the prevention of stent thrombosis.[13,14,20,21]

counts be obtained after starting ticlopidine. Other side-effects include rash (11.6%), diarrhea (20.7%), dyspepsia (10.4%), nausea (11.4%), liver dysfunction, and bronchiolitis obliterans organizing pneumonia.[22,23]

## Clopidogrel

Clopidogrel is a newer thienopyridine derivative related to ticlopidine. Its mechanism of action is similar and it is several times more potent than ticlopidine. Clopidogrel in combination with aspirin is equally efficacious as ticlopidine plus aspirin in preventing major adverse cardiac events (MACE) after stenting in the CLASSICS (Clopidogrel Aspirin Stent International Cooperative Study) trial (Table 11.1).[24] A meta-analysis of the randomized trials and registries comparing clopidogrel to ticlopidine in 13 955 patients showed MACE of 2 and 4% respectively. Thirty-day mortality was lower for clopidogrel compared to ticlopidine (0.5% vs 1.1%). The major advantage of clopidogrel over ticlopidine is its safety profile.[24] In 19 185 patients enrolled in the CAPRIE (Clopidogrel versus Aspirin in Patients at Risk of Ischemic Events) trial the incidence of neutropenia was 0.16%, diarrhea 4.5%, and skin rash 6.0% in the clopidogrel arm.[26] These data suggest that clopidogrel is better tolerated and has fewer side-effects compared to ticlopidine.

| Table 11.1. CLASSICS trial (*n* = 1020)[24] | ASA 325 mg/day + Plavix 75 mg | ASA 325 mg/day + Ticlid 250 mg | P value |
|---|---|---|---|
| Bleeding, neutropenia, thrombocytopenia, early discontinuation | 4.6% | 9.1% | 0.005 |
| Major adverse events (death, MI, TVR) | 1.5% | 0.9% | NS |

ASA, aspirin; MI, myocardial infarction; NS, non-significant; TVR, target vessel revascularization.

## Timing, loading dose, and duration of therapy

Pretreatment with clopidogrel improves patient outcomes. In the PCI-CURE (Clopidogrel in Unstable angina to prevent Recurrent Events, PCI substudy) trial patients treated with aspirin plus clopidogrel for a median of six days prior to intervention had lower incidence of cardiovascular death, MI, or urgent target vessel revascularization (TVR) at 30 days (4.5% vs 6.5% for the placebo).[27] In the real world most patients with non-ST elevation MI undergo revascularization within 4 to 48 hours; adequate time for pretreatment with clopidogrel may not exist.

The CREDO (Clopidogrel for the Reduction of Events During Observation) trial addressed this issue regarding pretreatment with clopidogrel in more than 2100 patients with a 300 mg loading dose of clopidogrel given 3 to 24 hours prior to catheterization.[27] All patients received aspirin plus clopidogrel 75 mg/day for a period of one year. At 28 days there was a trend toward reduction of MACE with clopidogrel compared to placebo (6.8% vs 8.3%). In a subset analysis, benefit is seen in patients who received clopidogrel $\geq$ 6 hours. In patients receiving the pretreatment dose of clopidogrel < 6 hours had no benefit. At one year the combined end-point of death, MI, and stroke was significantly reduced by loading and long-term treatment with clopidogrel (8.5% vs 11.5% with placebo; P = 0.02).

In the DES trials, the duration of antiplatelet therapy ranged from two months in the RAVEL trial to six months in the TAXUS (Taxol-eluting stent) trial. After DES implantation, double antiplatelet therapy should be continued for at least three months and preferably 6 to 12 months. The CREDO trial suggested that double antiplatelet therapy for at least one year confers benefits in terms of MI and death, in addition to protection against stent thrombosis.

## Anticoagulation

### Heparin

Intravenous unfractionated heparin is typically given during stent placement to prevent intraprocedural coronary thrombus leading to acute vessel closure.[29] Heparin monitoring is performed using the activated clotting time (ACT). A target ACT of 250 to 350 seconds is most often used in interventional practice today. Pooled data from six randomized trials showed that an ACT of 350 to 375 seconds was associated with the lowest ischemic events at seven days after intervention.[30] With the concomitant use of glycoprotein IIb/IIIa inhibitors the desired ACT is 200 to 250 seconds. Evidence for this comes from the ESPRIT (Enhanced Suppression of the Platelet IIb/IIIa Receptor with Integrilin Therapy) trial.[31] A weight-based heparin-dosing regimen (60 IU/kg) was used to achieve a target ACT of 200 to 300 seconds. In both the SIRIUS and TAXUS trials, unfractionated heparin in standard doses were used. There are no data regarding the use of low-molecular-weight heparin with DES.

## Direct thrombin inhibitors

The benefit of bivaluridin, a direct thrombin inhibitor, was defined in the REPLACE-2 (Randomized Evaluation in PCI Linking Angiomax to Reduced Clinical Events) trial.[32] In this trial, of the 6010 patients enrolled 85% received a stent. Patients were randomized to unfractionated heparin with planned glycoprotein IIb/IIIa inhibitors or bivaluridin with provisional glycoprotein IIb/IIIa inhibitors. The use of bivaluridin was associated with less bleeding (2.4% vs 4.1%) and was non-inferior to heparin for the end-points of death, MI, and urgent revascularization.

Bivaluridin is less dependent upon renal clearance than heparin and hence may have less bleeding in patients with renal insufficiency.[33] The loading dose of bivaluridin is 0.75 mg/kg i.v. followed by 1.75 mg/kg/hr infusion for the duration of the procedure up to four hours. There are limited data regarding the use of bivaluridin in DES implantation. Preliminary data from the ADEST (Angiomax and Drug-Eluting Stent) study showed that the use of bivaluridin with a SES is safe and effective compared to a BMS.

## Conclusion

The incidence of stent thrombosis with DES is comparable to that with BMS. Currently available DES have stent thrombosis rates less than 1% when optimally deployed and two antiplatelet agents are used for several months. Double antiplatelet therapy with aspirin plus clopidogrel/ticlopidine should be continued for a period of at least three months and ideally 6 to 12 months.

## References

1. Serruys PW, de Jaegere P, Kiemeneij F et al. A comparison of balloon expandable stent implantation with balloon angioplasty in patients with coronary artery disease. N Engl J Med 1994; 331: 489

2. Serruys PW, Strauss BH, Beatt KJ et al. Angiographic follow-up after placement of self-expanding coronary artery stent. N Engl J Med 1991; 324: 13–17

3. Mak KH, Belli G, Ellis S et al. Subacute stent thrombosis evolving issues and current concepts. J Am Coll Cardiol 1996; 27: 494–503

4. Fischman DL, Leon MB, Baim DS et al. A randomized comparison of coronary stent placement and balloon angioplasty in the treatment of coronary artery disease. N Engl J Med 1994; 331: 496

5. De Palma VA, Baierre B, Ford JW et al. Investigation of three surface properties of several metals and their relation to blood biocompatibility. J Biomed Mater Res 1972; 3: 37–75

6. Schatz RA, Palmaz JC, Joffre R et al. Ballon-expandable intracoronary stents in the adult dog. Circulation 1987; 76: 450–57

7. Gawaz M, Neumann FJ, Ott I et al. Changes in membrane glycoproteins of circulating platelets after coronary stent implantation. Heart 1996; 76: 166–72

8. Lefkovits J, Plow EF, Topol EJ. Platelet glycoprotein IIb/IIIa receptors in cardiovascular medicine. N Engl J Med 1995; 332: 1553–59

9. Hong MK, Mintz GS, Lee CW et al. Paclitaxel coating reduces in-stent intimal hyperplasia in human coronary arteries: a serial volumetric intravascular ultrasound analysis from the Asian Paclitaxel-Eluting Stent clinical Trial (ASPECT). Circulation 2003; 107: 517–20

10. Moses JW, Leon MB, Popma JJ et al. Sirolimus-eluting stents versus standard stents in patients with stenosis in a native coronary artery. N Engl J Med 2003; 349: 1315

11. Regar E, Serruys PW, Bode C et al. Angiographic findings of the multicenter Randomized Study With the Sirolimus-Eluting Bx Velocity Balloon-Expandable Stent (RAVEL): sirolimus-eluting stents inhibit restenosis irrespective of the vessel size. Circulation 2002; 106: 1949

12. Schofer J, Schluter M, Gershlick AH et al. Sirolimus-eluting stents for treatment of patients with long atherosclerotic lesions in small coronary arteries: double-blind, randomised controlled trial (E-SIRIUS). Lancet 2003; 362: 1093

13. Schuhlen H, Hadamitzky M, Walter H et al. Major benefit from antiplatelet therapy for patients at high risk for adverse cardiac events after coronary Palmaz-Schatz stent placement. Analysis of a prospective risk stratification protocol in the Intracoronary Stenting and Antithrombotic Regimen (ISAR) trial. Circulation 1997; 95: 2015

14. Leon MB, Baim DS, Popma JJ et al, for the Stent Anticoagulation Restenosis Study Investigators. A clinical trial comparing three antithrombotic-drug regimens after coronary artery stenting. N Engl J Med 1998; 339: 1665

15. Stone GW, Ellis SG, Cox DA et al. A polymer-based, paclitaxel-eluting stent in patients with coronary artery disease. N Engl J Med 2004; 350: 221

16. The Dutch TIA Trial Study Group. A comparison of low doses of aspirin (30 mg vs 283 mg a day) in patients after a transient ischemic attack or minor ischemic stroke. N Engl J Med 1991; 325: 1261–66

17. The SALT Collaborative Group. Swedish Aspirin Low-Dose Trial (SALT) of 75 mg aspirin as secondary prophylaxis after cerebrovascular ischaemic events. Lancet 1991; 338: 1345–49

18. Antiplatelet Trialists' Collaboration. Collaborative overview of randomized trials of antiplatelet therapy. I. Prevention of death, myocardial infarction and stroke by prolonged antiplatelet therapy in various categories of patients. BMJ 1994; 308: 81–106

19. Barnathan ES, Schwartz JS, Taylor L et al. Aspirin and dypiridamole in the prevention of acute coronary thrombosis complicating coronary angioplasty. Circulation 1987; 76: 124–34

20. Bertrand ME, Legrand V, Boland J et al. Randomized multicenter comparison of conventional anticoagulation versus antiplatelet therapy in unplanned and elective coronary stenting: The Full Anticoagulation versus Aspirin and Ticlopidine (FANTASTIC) study. Circulation 1998; 98: 1567

21. Urban P, Macaya C, Rupprecht H-J et al., for the MATTIS Investigators. Randomized evaluation of anticoagulation versus antiplatelet therapy after

coronary stent implantation in high-risk patients: The Multicenter Aspirin and Ticlopidine Trial after Intracoronary Stenting (MATTIS). Circulation 1998; 98: 2126

22. Hass WK, Easton DJ, Adams HP et al. A randomized trial comparing ticlopidine hydrochloride with aspirin for the prevention of stroke in high-risk patients. N Engl J Med 1989; 321: 501–507

23. Gent M, Blakely JA, Easton JD et al. The Canadian American Ticlopidine Study (CATS) in thromboembolic stroke. Lancet 1989; 1: 1215–20

24. Bertrand ME, Rupprecht HJ, Urban P et al. Double-blind study of the safety of clopidogrel with and without a loading dose in combination with aspirin compared with ticlopidine in combination with aspirin after coronary stenting: the clopidogrel aspirin stent international cooperative study (CLASSICS). Circulation 2000; 102: 624

25. Bhatt DL, Bertrand ME, Berger PB et al. Meta-analysis of randomized and registry comparisons of ticlopidine with clopidogrel after stenting. J Am Coll Cardiol 2002; 39: 9

26. CAPRIE Steering Committee. A randomized, blinded trial of clopidogrel versus aspirin in patients at risk of ischaemic events. Lancet 1996; 348: 1329–39

27. Mehta SR, Yusuf S, Peters RJ et al. Effects of pretreatment with clopidogrel and aspirin followed by long-term therapy in patients undergoing percutaneous coronary intervention: the PCI-CURE study. Lancet 2001; 358: 527

28. Steinhubl SR, Berger PB, Mann JT 3rd et al. Early and sustained dual oral antiplatelet therapy following percutaneous coronary intervention: a randomized controlled trial. JAMA 2002; 288: 2411

29. Popma JJ, Weitz J, Bittl JA et al. Antithrombotic therapy in patients undergoing coronary angioplasty. Chest 1998; 114: 728S

30. Chew DP, Bhatt DL, Lincoff AM et al. Defining the optimal activated clotting time during percutaneous coronary intervention: aggregate results from 6 randomized, controlled trials. Circulation 2001; 103: 961

31. Tolleson TR, O'Shea JC, Bittl JA et al. Relationship between heparin anticoagulation and clinical outcomes in coronary stent intervention. Observations from the ESPRIT trial. J Am Coll Cardiol 2003; 41: 386

32. Lincoff AM, Bittl JA, Harrington RA et al. Bivalirudin and provisional glycoprotein IIb/IIIa blockade compared with heparin and planned glycoprotein IIb/IIIa blockade during percutaneous coronary intervention: REPLACE-2 randomized trial. JAMA 2003; 289: 853

33. Chew DP, Bhatt DL, Kimball W et al. Bivalirudin provides increasing benefit with decreasing renal function: a meta-analysis of randomized trials. Am J Cardiol 2003; 92: 919

# 12. Optimal Deployment Strategies for Drug-Eluting Stents

## Georges A Feghali and Bahij N Khuri

### Background

The early drug-eluting stent (DES) trials followed narrow enrollment criteria and showed a significant reduction in the restenosis rate compared to bare metal stents (BMS).[1–5] However, it is unclear whether DES placement outside of the clinical trials' criteria and across a broader spectrum of lesion and patient subsets will result in the same single digit restenosis rate. It is important to realize that optimal deployment strategies and techniques used in these early trials, in addition to the immunosuppressive and antiproliferative coatings applied to the surface of coronary stents, contributed to the favorable angiographic and clinical results.

### Bifurcation lesions

Bifurcation lesions have traditionally been the 'Achilles' heel' of interventional cardiology. Difficulties involving side-branch access and plaque shifting have resulted in the development of techniques to stent both the main (mother) and side (daughter) branches. Bifurcation lesions are classified according to lesion location (Figure 12.1) and by the angulation between main and side branches into 'Y' (<90°) or 'T' (90°) configurations.[6]

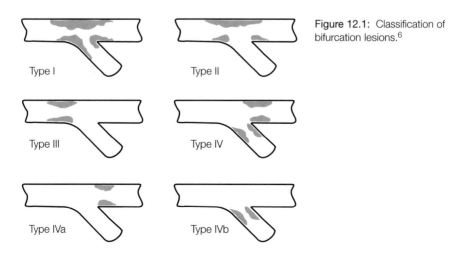

Type I  Type II  Type III  Type IV  Type IVa  Type IVb

**Figure 12.1:** Classification of bifurcation lesions.[6]

## Main vessel stenting and side-branch balloon angioplasty

This technique consists of placing a stent into the main vessel, across the ostium of the side-branch, followed by balloon angioplasty of the side-branch lesion through the struts of the main vessel stent. Typically, kissing balloons are not performed if the side-branch flow is not impaired or there is a mild stenosis in a side-branch.

## Main vessel and side-branch stenting

If it is necessary to place a second stent into the side-branch because of recoil or failure of balloon dilation, then one of several techniques may be considered (Figure 12.2):

- Stent implantation in the side-branch followed by stenting of the main vessel. The pitfall of this technique is incomplete coverage of the ostium of the side-branch. A modified technique – the 'crush technique' – provides a possible solution to this problem.[7,8]
- Stent implantation from the proximal to distal main vessel across the ostium of the side-branch followed by another stent from the proximal main vessel toward the side-branch – this technique is known as the 'culotte' or 'trousers' technique.[9]
- Simultaneous stent implantation at the ostium of the main vessel and side-branch followed by implantation of a third stent at the 'carina' if necessary.[10]

The drawback of stent implantation in the main and side branches has been the increased restenosis rate in the side-branch. Currently, stent placement into the main branch and balloon angioplasty with provisional stenting of the side-branch is the preferred technique to treat bifurcation lesions.[11-14] In fact, stenting both vessels has shown to be associated with a higher restenosis rate and target lesion revascularization (TLR) compared to stenting the main vessel and only balloon angioplasty of the side-branch.[11,12]

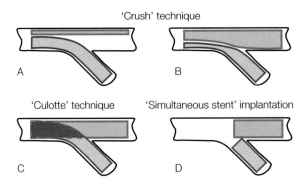

'Crush' technique

A          B

'Culotte' technique          'Simultaneous stent' implantation

C          D

Figure 12.2: (a and b) 'Crush' technique. (c) 'Culotte' technique. (d) 'Simultaneous stenting'.[11-14]

In a recent report, the implantation of DES in both vessels was associated with a 5.7% main vessel restenosis rate and 19% target vessel failure (TVF).[13] The high TVF was the result of high incidence of side-branch restenosis and stent thrombosis. In another report, stent implantation in the main vessel followed with provisional side-branch stenting appears to be the preferred technique to treat bifurcation lesions (Table 12.1).[14]

## Spot stenting versus complete coverage stenting

The RAVEL trial (RAndomised, double-blind study with the sirolimus-eluting Bx VELocity™ balloon-expandable stent in the treatment of patients with de-novo native coronary artery lesions) was the first randomized double-blind DES trial, which signaled the beginning of a new era in coronary interventions.[2] This study enrolled patients with single discreet lesions with an average lesion length of 9.6 ± 3.33 mm and reference vessel diameter (RVD) of 2.6 ± 0.54 mm. The six-month restenosis rate and TLR were both 0%. However, this absence of restenosis was not observed in the SIRIUS trial (SIRollmUS-coated Bx Velocity™ stent) (Figure 12.3).[3] The higher restenosis rate in SIRIUS was the result of higher-risk patients (diabetics, previous myocardial infarction, more complex lesions (longer length), and longer angiographic follow-up (nine months vs six months in RAVEL).

However, the differences in stent implantation technique (balloon size for pre- and post-dilation, stent length/lesion length ratio) may also have contributed to the restenosis discrepancies. RAVEL's protocol prohibited investigators from direct stenting, encouraged the use of shorter balloons for pre- and post-dilation to prevent proximal and distal edge injuries, and encouraged longer stents (stent length/lesion length ratio 2.2 for RAVEL vs 1.6 for SIRIUS) to ensure a full coverage of lesions and/or balloon-injured segments. The increased incidence of restenosis at the proximal stent edge observed in SIRIUS (Figure 12.4) may have been the result of incomplete

| Table 12.1. Restenosis rate according to technique | | | |
|---|---|---|---|
| Technique | Stent and kissing balloon | T stent and kissing balloon | Modified Y stents |
| Patient (n) | 13 | 13 | 16 |
| RR in SB (%) | 7.7 | 23.1 | 18.8 |
| RR in MB (%) | 0 | 0 | 6.2 |
| RR in MB and SB (%) | 0 | 7.7 | 6.2 |
| RR (%) | 7.7 | 30.8 | 31.2 |

MB, main branch; RR, restenosis rate; SB, side-branch.

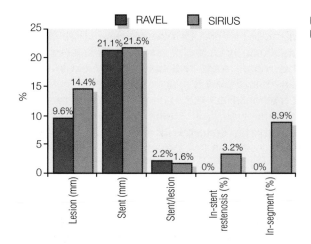

**Figure 12.3:** DES results: RAVEL versus SIRIUS.[2,3]

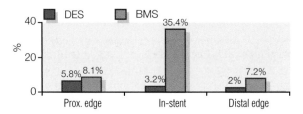

**Figure 12.4:** SIRIUS trial: peri-stent analysis.[3]

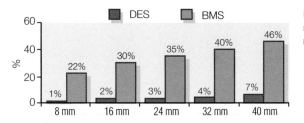

**Figure 12.5:** SIRIUS trial: stent length and in-stent restenosis.[3]

lesion coverage. Drug-eluting stents have disrupted the established direct relationship between BMS length and restenosis (Figure 12.5). The placement of longer DES in RAVEL resulted in better or more complete lesion coverage and therefore a lower proximal stent edge restenosis rate.

The E-SIRIUS (European) and C-SIRIUS trials enrolled patients at higher risk for restenosis. The restenosis rate in the control group of E-SIRIUS was 42.3% compared to a lower rate (26.6%) in the control group of RAVEL and yet the treatment groups showed a very low incidence of in-segment restenosis (ISR): 5.9% and 2.3%, respectively.[15,16] Both of these recent studies allowed direct stenting and encouraged the use of shorter balloons for pre- and post-dilation, more than one stent to ensure complete lesion coverage (⩾2 stents implanted in 40% of patients in C-SIRIUS), and overlapping stents by 2–4 mm to avoid gaps. This stent placement technique followed in E-SIRIUS and C-SIRIUS may have been behind the favorable outcomes observed in these trials (Table 12.2).

The ongoing STELLAR trial is designed to answer questions regarding optimal DES deployment. Until then, the preferred strategies for DES deployment should include shorter balloons for pre- and post-dilation, complete lesion coverage of lesion and/or balloon-injured segment (⩾2 stents if necessary), and direct stenting.

## Diameter sizing

In theory, the apposition of DES to the vessel wall should ensure better drug delivery to target cells. However, the high incidence of incomplete stent apposition detected in RAVEL did not have an adverse effect on outcome.

| Table 12.2. Characteristics of SIRIUS, E-SIRIUS, and C-SIRIUS[3,15,16] | | | |
|---|---|---|---|
| | *SIRIUS* (n = 1058)* | *E-SIRIUS* (n = 352)† | *C-SIRIUS* (n = 100)‡ |
| Age (years) | 62 | 62 | 60 |
| Diabetes (%) | 26 | 19 | 24 |
| Prior MI (%) | 31 | 41 | 48 |
| Lesion length (mm) | 14.4 | 14.9 | 14.5 |
| RVD (mm) | 2.8 | 2.6 | 2.65 |
| Stent length (mm) | 21.5 | 23 | 23.8 |
| Stent to lesion ratio | 1.6 | 1.7 | 1.8 |
| Patients with overlapping stents (%) | 28.5 | 34 | 40 |
| Direct stenting (%) | 0 | 26 | 31 |
| In-lesion RR (%) | 8.9 | 5.9 | 2.3 |
| In-stent RR (%) | 3.2 | 3.9 | 0 |
| Proximal edge RR (%) | 5.8 | 2.1 | 2.3 |
| Distal edge RR (%) | 2.0 | 1.3 | 0 |
| TLR (%) | 3.9 | 4 | 4 |

*703 patients were available for the eight-month angiographic follow-up.
†308 patients were available for the eight-month angiographic follow-up.
‡88 patients were available for the eight-month angiographic follow-up.
MI, myocardial infarction; RR, restenosis rate; RVD, reference vessel diameter; TLR, target lesion revascularization.

Patients with incomplete stent apposition by intravascular ultrasound (IVUS) were followed for 12 months with no evidence of adverse outcomes compared to those with complete DES apposition.[17]

The angiographic goal for stent implantation in E-SIRIUS and C-SIRIUS was to expand the DES slightly more than the RVD. The deployment goal in RAVEL and SIRIUS was to obtain a residual stenosis below 20% and below 30%, respectively. It appears safe and efficacious to choose a nominal stent sized to a RVD ratio of 1:1 and, if necessary, post-dilate in order to obtain a stent segment slightly larger than the RVD or a residual stenosis below 20%.

## Optimal overlap

In order to avoid gaps between stents, investigators in SIRIUS, E-SIRIUS and C-SIRIUS allowed stent overlap of 2–4 mm (28.5%, 34%, and 40%, respectively). This practice appears to be safe and resulted in a very low restenosis rate (3.2%, 3.9%, and 0%, respectively).

Intravascular ultrasound was performed to evaluate the effect of DES overlap for ISR.[18] At the one-year follow-up, changes in intravascular measurements within the overlapped segments were not different. The effect of paclitaxel on neointimal hyperplasia is dose-dependent with a narrower therapeutic window compared to sirolimus.[19,20] The TAXUS trials have demonstrated safety and efficacy for de-novo lesions less than 28 mm in length amenable to single stent coverage.[4,5] However, the safety of overlapping TAXUS stents has not been established. An ongoing trial, TAXUS V, will provide answers regarding the use of multiple overlapping TAXUS stents.

## Upsizing small stents for larger vessels

The post-dilation of bare metal stents with balloons > 0.25 mm larger than the stent's nominal size has been shown to be safe and to improve acute luminal gain.[21–23] The post-dilation of DES may lead to disruption of mechanical and biological properties of the polymer which could adversely affect outcome. However, minimal post-dilation of DES with slightly over-sized balloons (balloon to stent ratio 1.1:1) in RAVEL did not have an unfavorable effect on outcome.

The RESEARCH registry demonstrated that over-dilation of sirolimus-eluting stents with > 1 mm over-sized balloons, was safe and effective.[17] The reported restenosis rate, TVR, and TLR (7.7%, 6%, and 4.5% respectively) are in agreement with the results of other DES studies. In their registry, only one (1.5%) patient underwent emergency bypass surgery due to coronary dissection, and 3 (4.4%) patients died (only one from a cardiac cause).

## The role of intravascular ultrasound

Intravascular ultrasound (IVUS) has played a central role in explaining disease mechanisms and establishing new techniques in interventional cardiology.

However, the role of IVUS in optimizing coronary stent deployment remains controversial. It has been able to demonstrate incomplete stent deployment after angiography-guided stenting in a minority of patients.[24,25] Subsequent randomized controlled trials (SIPS, RESIST, and OPTICUS) have shown that IVUS-guided stenting was equivalent to angiographically guided stenting in terms of composite end-point of death and MI, as well as binary restenosis.[25–27]

A reduction in TLR in patients with small vessels, saphenous vein graft lesions, and larger vessels with long lesions has been shown in several trials. A recent meta-analysis[28] of randomized controlled trials and registries has shown no impact of IVUS-guided stenting on composite end-point (death and MI) when compared to angiographically guided stenting (Figure 12.6).[28] However, when registries are accounted for there was a statistically significant reduction in binary restenosis in favor of IVUS-guided stenting (Figure 12.7).

## Conclusion

Observations made in the early DES trials have demonstrated the importance of stent deployment technique for achieving optimal clinical results. The STELLAR trial is designed to provide answers to questions regarding the optimal DES deployment techniques. At the present time, DES strategies have evolved to recognize that bifurcation lesions continue to pose

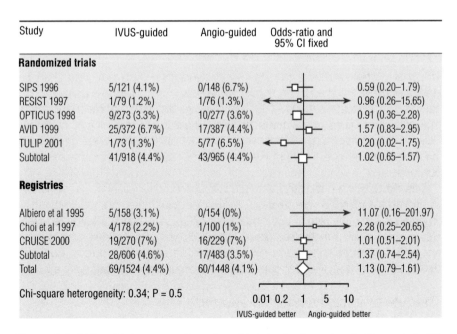

| Study | IVUS-guided | Angio-guided | Odds-ratio and 95% CI fixed | |
| --- | --- | --- | --- | --- |
| **Randomized trials** | | | | |
| SIPS 1996 | 5/121 (4.1%) | 0/148 (6.7%) | | 0.59 (0.20–1.79) |
| RESIST 1997 | 1/79 (1.2%) | 1/76 (1.3%) | | 0.96 (0.26–15.65) |
| OPTICUS 1998 | 9/273 (3.3%) | 10/277 (3.6%) | | 0.91 (0.36–2.28) |
| AVID 1999 | 25/372 (6.7%) | 17/387 (4.4%) | | 1.57 (0.83–2.95) |
| TULIP 2001 | 1/73 (1.3%) | 5/77 (6.5%) | | 0.20 (0.02–1.75) |
| Subtotal | 41/918 (4.4%) | 43/965 (4.4%) | | 1.02 (0.65–1.57) |
| **Registries** | | | | |
| Albiero et al 1995 | 5/158 (3.1%) | 0/154 (0%) | | 11.07 (0.16–201.97) |
| Choi et al 1997 | 4/178 (2.2%) | 1/100 (1%) | | 2.28 (0.25–20.65) |
| CRUISE 2000 | 19/270 (7%) | 16/229 (7%) | | 1.01 (0.51–2.01) |
| Subtotal | 28/606 (4.6%) | 17/483 (3.5%) | | 1.37 (0.74–2.54) |
| Total | 69/1524 (4.4%) | 60/1448 (4.1%) | | 1.13 (0.79–1.61) |

Chi-square heterogeneity: 0.34; P = 0.5

0.01  0.2   1   5   10

IVUS-guided better          Angio-guided better

Figure 12.6: IVUS-guided versus angiography-guided stenting (reproduced with permission).[28]

| Study | IVUS-guided | Angio-guided | Odds-ratio and 95% CI fixed | |
|---|---|---|---|---|
| **Randomized trials** | | | | |
| SIPS 1996 | 48/166 (29%) | 66/190 (34.7%) | | 0.76 (0.49–1.20) |
| RESIST 1997 | 16/71 (22.5%) | 21/73 (28.7%) | | 0.72 (0.34–1.53) |
| OPTICUS 1998 | 56/229 (24.4%) | 52/228 (22.8%) | | 1.10 (0.71–1.69) |
| TULIP 2001 | 15/73 (20.5%) | 28/77 (36.4%) | | 0.45 (0.02–0.94) |
| Subtotal | 135/539 (25%) | 167/568 (29%) | | 0.81 (0.62–1.06) |
| **Registries** | | | | |
| Albiero et al 1995 | 29/158 (18.3%) | 40/154 (26%) | | 0.64 (0.37–1.10) |
| Blasini et al 1997 | 22/105 (20.9%) | 32/107 (29.9%) | | 0.62 (0.33–1.16) |
| Subtotal | 51/263 (19%) | 72/261 (27.5%) | | 0.63 (0.42–0.95) |
| Total | 186/802 (23%) | 239/829 (28.8%) | | 0.73 (0.60–0.94) |

Chi-square heterogeneity: 0.36; P = 0.1

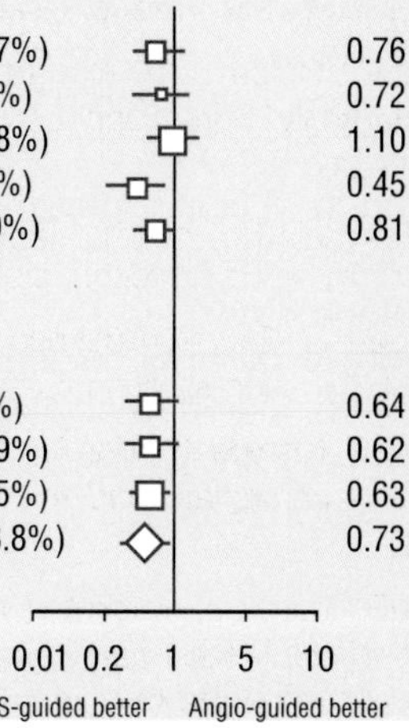

0.01 0.2 1 5 10

IVUS-guided better    Angio-guided better

Figure 12.7: IVUS-guided stenting: restenosis (reproduced with permission).[28]

challenges, that complete lesion coverage is important, that there is no restenosis penalty for longer stent use, that DES to vessel sizing should be 1:1 with the role of overdilation of undersized stents, and that IVUS-guided stenting requires further investigation.

## References

1. Sousa JE, Costa MA, Abizaid AC et al. Sustained suppression of neointimal proliferation by sirolimus-eluting stents: one-year angiographic and intravascular ultrasound follow-up. Circulation 2001; 104(17): 2007–11

2. Morice MC, Serruys PW, Sousa JE et al. A randomized comparison of a sirolimus-eluting stent with a standard stent for coronary revascularization. N Engl J Med 2002; 346(23): 1773–80

3. Moses JW, Leon MB, Popma JJ et al. Sirolimus-eluting stents versus standard stents in patients with stenosis in a native coronary artery. N Engl J Med 2003; 349(14): 1315–23

4. Colombo A, Drzewiecki J, Banning A et al. Randomized study to assess the effectiveness of slow- and moderate-release polymer-based paclitaxel-eluting stents for coronary artery lesions. Circulation 2003; 108(7): 788–94

5. Stone GW, Ellis SG, Cox DA et al. A polymer-based, paclitaxel-eluting stent in patients with coronary artery disease. N Engl J Med 2004; 350(3): 221–31

6. Di Mario C, Airoldi F, Reimers B et al. Bifurcational stenting. Semin Interv Cardiol 1998; 3(2): 65–76

7. Louvard Y, Lefevre T, Morice MC. Percutaneous coronary intervention for bifurcation coronary disease. Heart 2004; 90(6): 713–22

8. Kobayashi Y, Colombo A, Akiyama T et al. Modified "T" stenting: a technique for kissing stents in bifurcational coronary lesion. Catheter Cardiovasc Diagn 1998; 43(3): 323–26

9. Chevalier B, Glatt B, Royer T et al. Placement of coronary stents in bifurcation lesions by the "culotte" technique. Am J Cardiol 1998; 82(8): 943–49

10. Schampaert E, Fort S, Adelman AG et al. The V-stent: a novel technique for coronary bifurcation stenting. Catheter Cardiovasc Diagn 1996; 39(3): 320–26

11. Yamashita T, Nishida T, Adamian MG et al. Bifurcation lesions: two stents versus one stent – immediate and follow-up results. J Am Coll Cardiol 2000; 35(5): 1145–51

12. Cervinka P, Stasek J, Pleskot M et al. Treatment of coronary bifurcation lesions by stent implantation only in parent vessel and angioplasty in sidebranch: immediate and long-term outcome. J Invasive Cardiol 2002; 14(12): 735–40

13. Colombo A, Moses JW, Morice MC et al. Randomized study to evaluate sirolimus-eluting stents implanted at coronary bifurcation lesions. Circulation 2004; 109(10): 1244–49

14. Colombo A, Louvard Y, Raghu C et al. Sirolimus-eluting stents in bifurcation lesions: six-month angiographic results according to the implantation technique (abstract). J Am Coll Cardiol 2003; 41: 53A

15. Schampaert E, Cohen EA, Schluter M et al. The Canadian study of the sirolimus-eluting stent in the treatment of patients with long de novo lesions in small native coronary arteries (C-SIRIUS). J Am Coll Cardiol 2004; 43(6): 1110–15

16. Schofer J, Schluter M, Gershlick AH et al. Sirolimus-eluting stents for treatment of patients with long atherosclerotic lesions in small coronary arteries: double-blind, randomised controlled trial (E-SIRIUS). Lancet 2003; 362(9390): 1093–99

17. Saia F, Lemos PA, Arampatzis CA et al. Clinical and angiographic outcomes after overdilatation of undersized sirolimus-eluting stents with largely oversized balloons: an observational study. Catheter Cardiovasc Interv 2004; 61(4): 455–60

18. Munoz JS, Abizaid A, Mintz GS et al. Intravascular ultrasound study of effects of overlapping sirolimus-eluting stents. Am J Cardiol 2004; 93(4): 470–73

19. Kornowski R, Hong MK, Ragheb AO et al. Slow-release Taxol-coated GR-II stents reduce neointimal formation in porcine coronary in-stent restenosis model (abstract). Circulation 1997; 96 (Suppl): I-341

20. Lau KW, Mak KH, Hung JS et al. Clinical impact of stent construction and design in percutaneous coronary intervention. Am Heart J 2004; 147(5): 764–73

21. Stone GW, Hodgson JM, St Goar FG et al. Improved procedural results of coronary angioplasty with intravascular ultrasound-guided balloon sizing: the CLOUT Pilot Trial. Clinical Outcomes With Ultrasound Trial (CLOUT) Investigators. Circulation 1997; 95(8): 2044–52

22. Schroeder S, Baumbach A, Haase KK et al. Reduction of restenosis by vessel size adapted percutaneous transluminal coronary angioplasty using intravascular ultrasound. Am J Cardiol 1999; 83(6): 875–79

23. Johansson B, Allared M, Borgencrantz B et al. Standardized angiographically guided over-dilatation of stents using high-pressure technique optimize results without increasing risks. J Inv Cardiol 2002; 14(5): 221–26

24. Colombo A, Hall P, Nakamura S et al. Intracoronary stenting without anticoagulation accomplished with intravascular ultrasound guidance. Circulation 1995; 91(6): 1676–88

25. Frey AW, Hodgson JM, Muller C et al. Ultrasound-guided strategy for provisional stenting with focal balloon combination catheter: results from the randomized Strategy for Intracoronary Ultrasound-guided PTCA and Stenting (SIPS) trial. Circulation 2000; 102(20): 2497–502

26. Schiele F, Meneveau N, Vuillemenot A et al. Impact of intravascular ultrasound guidance in stent deployment on 6-month restenosis rate: a multicenter, randomized study comparing two strategies – with and without intravascular ultrasound guidance. RESIST Study Group. REStenosis after Ivus guided STenting. J Am Coll Cardiol 1998; 32(2): 320–28

27. Mudra H, di Mario C, de Jaegere P et al. Randomized comparison of coronary stent implantation under ultrasound or angiographic guidance to reduce stent restenosis (OPTICUS Study). Circulation 2001; 104(12): 1343–49

28. Casella G, Klauss V, Ottani F et al. Impact of intravascular ultrasound-guided stenting on long-term clinical outcome: a meta-analysis of available studies comparing intravascular ultrasound-guided and angiographically guided stenting. Catheter Cardiovasc Interv 2003; 59(3): 314–21

# PART V

# COST–BENEFIT ANALYSIS AND FUTURE STRATEGIES FOR DRUG-ELUTING STENTS

# 13. Cost Analysis for Coronary Drug-Eluting Stents

## John P Reilly

## Introduction

Drug-eluting stents (DES) have revolutionized interventional cardiology, significantly reducing restenosis, one of the most difficult obstacles that remain in treating obstructive coronary disease.[1–3] This is one of a handful of technologies that has achieved greater efficacy without increased risk to the patient. The enthusiasm with which this technology was anticipated, and subsequently embraced, has been tempered only by the significant increase in cost.

The Palmaz–Schatz stent was approved for use in coronary arteries in 1994. Initial trials demonstrated coronary stents' significantly lower restenosis rates compared to percutaneous transluminal coronary angioplasty (PTCA).[4] Stent implantation was associated with increased cost as stents were more expensive than balloon catheters. Patients were placed on an intense anticoagulation regimen which included intravenous heparin and dextran, oral aspirin, and warfarin therapy. Hospital stays were prolonged in order to find the appropriate warfarin dose, and due to bleeding complications. Despite the increased cost associated with stent implantation, the Healthcare Financing Administration, now known as the Center for Medicare and Medicaid Services (CMS), did not approve a separate reimbursement code until 1996.

Familiar with this history, industry incorporated cost-effectiveness analyses into the design of their DES clinical trials in the USA. Despite this proactive approach, which was intended to avoid the gap between stent approval and reimbursement, an uncertainty remains about the impact of DES on the economy of health care.

## Cost-effectiveness

Simply defined, cost-effectiveness analysis compares the cost of a proposed technology or strategy to the benefits of that technology or strategy. An incremental cost-effectiveness ratio is the difference in cost of a new technology divided by the incremental benefit of that technology. In health care, incremental benefit is usually measured in quality adjusted life years. Restenosis, however, being a relatively slow predictable process, rarely results in myocardial infarction (MI) or death. Repeat revascularization due to restenosis impacts on quality of life, but little data exist to quantify the magnitude of this impact. Interventional cardiology has developed a convention for examining technologies and strategies designed to reduce restenosis by comparing costs in US dollars to repeat revascularizations avoided. The US market has accepted a cost-effectiveness ratio of less than $10 000 per revascularization avoided for intracoronary brachytherapy and stent implantation versus PTCA.[5,6]

Greenberg et al. performed an analysis to create a model for patients undergoing single-vessel percutaneous coronary intervention (PCI). Data included one-year outcomes on 7000 patients after bare metal stent (BMS) implantation. Costs of PCI, its complications, and treatment for restenosis were based on 3000 patients pooled from several multicenter trials. They assumed a BMS restenosis rate of 14%, an 80% reduction in target vessel revascularization (TVR) with DES an incremental cost of $2000 per DES, and an average of 1.4 stents per procedure. This model predicts that over two years, the overall costs would be $900 more per patient in whom a DES was implanted compared to BMS. This represents an incremental cost-effectiveness ratio of $7000 per repeat revascularization avoided. If any of the assumptions made for this model are changed, then the cost-effectiveness ratio must be adjusted, i.e. if the relative costs of DES and BMS changed, or if fewer stents per procedure are used. In patients whose predicted TVR rate with BMS is greater than 20%, implantation of DES would be cost-saving, and in patients whose TVR rates with BMS are greater than 12%, implantation of DES would be cost-effective.[7,8]

Restenosis rates for BMS may be predicted accurately based on clinical and angiographic criteria (Table 13.1). The presence of diabetes, smaller vessel diameter and longer lesions predict greater restenosis. The predicted restenosis rates for most diabetics make implantation of DES cost-effective except in vessels $\geq$ 4 mm, or in 3.5 mm vessels with lesions < 25 mm in length. In non-diabetic patients, most lesions in vessels $\leq$ 3.0 mm represent cost-effective opportunities for DES implantation.[9]

## Reimbursement and diagnosis-related groups

The CMS establishes diagnosis-related groups (DRGs) to determine hospital reimbursement based on diagnosis rather than actual costs. This system is meant to remove the incentive for unnecessary tests and prolonged hospital stays. After some delay, the CMS established two DRGs distinct from PTCA to cover BMS implantation (with and without MI). In October 2003 the incremental reimbursement for DES (with and without MI) compared to BMS was established as $1650.[10]

Currently, the incremental cost of DES over BMS is approximately $1600 to $1800; the DRG for DES just covers the cost of one additional stent. However, the conservative estimate of mean DES usage is 1.4 stents per

**Table 13.1. Estimated risk of restenosis with bare metal stents**

| Diabetes | Lesion length | | | | |
|---|---|---|---|---|---|
| Vessel diameter (mm) | 10 mm | 15 mm | 20 mm | 25 mm | 30 mm |
| 2.5 | 23% | 26% | 29% | 31% | 34% |
| 3.0 | 15% | 17% | 20% | 22% | 24% |
| 3.5 | 10% | 11% | 13% | 15% | 16% |
| 4.0 | 6% | 7% | 8% | 9% | 10% |
| No diabetes | Lesion length | | | | |
| Vessel Diameter (mm) | 10 mm | 15 mm | 20 mm | 25 mm | 30 mm |
| 2.5 | 18% | 20% | 22% | 25% | 27% |
| 3.0 | 11% | 13% | 15% | 17% | 18% |
| 3.5 | 7% | 8% | 9% | 11% | 12% |
| 4.0 | 4% | 5% | 5% | 7% | 7% |

Shaded areas represent advantages for drug-eluting stents.

procedure, with some estimates as high as 1.7 to 2.0 DES per procedure. Given these costs and stent usage, current Medicare reimbursement rates decrease hospital profits. Actual payer mix will determine the profitability of revascularization (Table 13.2).[10]

## Impact on coronary bypass surgery

From 1998 to 2001, there was a steady increase in percutaneous revascularization among Medicare beneficiaries from 72 per 10 000 to 89.3 per 10 000. Over that time, the number of coronary artery bypass graft (CABG) surgeries decreased from 51 per 10 000 to 49.2 per 10 000. This increase in percutaneous intervention coincides with improvement in BMS technology (e.g. deliverability) as stent procedures increased from 50.9 per 10 000 in 1998 to 72 per 10 000 in 2001. In the US 90% of Medicare patients undergoing CABG have multivessel disease.[10] In the BARI trial, the difference between the CABG arm and those undergoing multivessel PTCA was in the rate of repeat revascularization. Mortality and MI rates were not different.[11] Similarly, in the ARTS trial, which randomized 1205 patients to multivessel BMS implantation versus CABG, death (3.7% vs 4.6%), cerebrovascular accident (3.3% vs 3.3%), and MI (7.3% vs 5.7%) were not different between the two groups. At three years, 29.2% of the patients in the stent arm underwent repeat revascularization compared to only 7.3% of those in the surgery arm.[12]

Table 13.2. Cost estimate for DES in a program with 350 CABG and 650 stents per year

|  | Industry assumptions | Worst-case assumptions |
| --- | --- | --- |
| Payer mix | 50% CMS/41% insured/9% other | 50% CMS/41% insured/9% other |
| Stent with AMI | 1.5 stents/case | 2.0 stents/case |
| Stent without AMI | 1.7 stents/case | 2.0 stents/case |
| CABG migration DES | 10% | 50% |
| PTCA migration DES | 15% | 80% |
| Reduction readmission | 25% | 80% |
| BMS cost | $1200 | $1200 |
| DES cost | $3200 | $3200 |
| Stent with AMI | 1.5 stents/case | 2.0 stents/case |
| Stent without AMI | 1.7 stents/case | 2.0 stents/case |
| Incremental cost/case | $3000 | $4000 |
| Gain/loss per case | ($164) | ($2980) |
| Total | ($164 000) | ($2 980 000) |

AMI, acute myocardial infarction; BMS, bare metal stent; CABG, coronary artery bypass graft; CMS, Center for Medicare and Medicaid Services; DES, drug-eluting stent; PTCA, percutaneous transluminal coronary angioplasty.

Assuming that the majority of the repeat revascularization seen in these trials is due to restenosis, we would expect that DES would make the outcomes in these two groups even more comparable. In one retrospective analysis, 196 consecutive angiograms of patients referred for CABG prior to the availability of DES were reviewed; 21% of the patients would not have been referred for CABG had DES been available. Chronic total occlusions, the presence of left main stenoses, and concomitant valvular disease requiring surgical repair predicted referral for surgery.[13] According to estimates made by the Centers for Disease Control (CDC), based on data from short-stay hospitals in the USA, 305 000 patients underwent CABG in 2001. This suggests that as many as 64 000 fewer patients in the USA might be referred for CABG due to the availability of DES.

## Impact on hospital revenue

Clark et al. modeled the impact on hospitals of the various revascularization strategies. BMS implantation yields a profit of $285; the average hospital lost $1389 per initial DES patient when all sources of payment were considered.[14] As the average number of stents per patient increases, hospital profits decrease. Hospital profits decrease as the percentage of private payers decreased.[10] CABG generated $1283 in profit for hospitals. With DES available, it is anticipated that a greater number of patients will undergo stent implantation, as has been true for the past five years with BMS. Hospitals will generate less revenue as more patients are converted from a relatively high profit margin procedure (CABG) to a lower profit margin procedure (stent implantation).[10] According to this same report, hospital profits will be maintained until 1.8 DES per patient are implanted and the conversion of BMS and CABG are over 80% and 15%, respectively.[14]

Cardiac catheterization laboratories have come to expect that 15% of the stents implanted will develop restenosis, necessitating repeat procedures within the first year. As a greater percentage of DES are implanted, the restenosis rate will fall to 5%.[1-3] These laboratories can expect a reduction in procedure volume, specifically a reduction in interventional volume, as the restenosis rate falls in patients treated with DES.

On the other hand, over the past few years, with BMS interventional cardiologists have implanted stents in increasingly complex patients. A greater number of patients with diabetes and patients with multivessel disease are treated with stent implantation rather than being referred for CABG. Given an improved device, interventional cardiologists will continue to expand the population of patients referred for percutaneous intervention. Approximately 90% of patients in the Medicare database are referred for CABG for multivessel disease. When technically feasible, an even greater number of patients with diabetes and patients with multivessel disease and small vessel disease will be treated in the catheterization laboratory rather than the operating room. Currently, 20% of patients undergoing stent implantation have multivessel disease, and this is expected to increase to 29% with DES adoption.[10] As more complex patients are treated percutaneously, a greater percentage of these procedures will be performed using ancillary devices and drugs such as intravascular ultrasound, embolic protection devices, and glycoprotein IIb/IIIa inhibitors, increasing the costs of a low-profit procedure.[10]

Whether treatment of left main disease will continue to require referral for surgical revascularization is unclear. Treatment of left main disease with CABG, particularly in the presence of left ventricular dysfunction, results in improved survival compared to medical therapy.[15] The major limitation of BMS in left main disease was not procedural success but restenosis. With DES available, will interventional cardiologists recommend stent implantation for left main disease? The answer remains unknown.

## Conclusion

The interpretation of the economic impact of DES depends upon one's perspective. From the hospital's point of view, DES will increase the cost of percutaneous intervention, with only a slight increase in reimbursement, and decrease the number of profitable CABG procedures performed.

Cardiologists will likely refer 20% fewer patients for CABG,[13] a procedure with a higher profit margin. From the payer's perspective, despite the increase in upfront costs, DES will result in a net reduction in expenditure. Fewer repeat revascularizations will be required and fewer patients will be referred for high-cost CABG. Lemos et al. estimated that 1 000 000 PCI are performed annually, 80% of which involve stent implantation. Assuming 100% DES use, and 1.5 stents per patient at an increased cost of $2000 per stent, there would be an increase of $2.4 billion per year in the USA. With a 15% reduction in reinterventions, saving $10 000 to $12 000 for percutaneous procedures and $20 000 to $30 000 for CABG, the cost of DES will be offset by $900 million per year. This adjustment for reduced restenosis would mean that the increase in costs in the USA would be roughly $1.5 billion per year.[16]

Drug-eluting stents will result in an increase in overall costs for US health care and reduce profits for hospitals. From the patient's perspective, DES implantation is a cost-effective strategy to reduce restenosis, although some patients would choose a DES over a BMS at any cost. Drug-eluting stent implantation is less than $10 000 per revascularization avoided, which has been considered an acceptable ratio for other strategies intended to reduce the need for revascularization, such as intracoronary brachytherapy.[5,6] Physicians must be guided by evidence from clinical trials, implanting DES in those patients whose risk of restenosis is greater than 12%.[17] To prevent hospitals from discouraging or limiting DES implantation, the CMS should consider adjusting the DRGs for DES reimbursement to more accurately reflect the increased cost of these procedures.

## References

1. Grube E, Silber S, Hauptmann KE et al. TAXUS I: six- and twelve-month results from a randomized, double-blind trial on a slow-release paclitaxel-eluting stent for de novo coronary lesions. Circulation 2003; 107: 38–42

2. Moses J, Leon M, Popma J et al. A multicenter randomized clinical study of the sirolimus-eluting stent in native coronary lesions: clinical outcomes. In: American Heart Association Scientific Sessions. Chicago, IL. Circulation; 2002: II-392

3. Leon M, Moses J, Popma J et al. A multicenter randomized clinical study of the sirolimus-eluting stent in native coronary lesions: angiographic results. In: Circulation (Suppl II) 393. Chicago, IL. American Heart Association Scientific Sessions; 2002: 393

4. Serruys PW, de Jaegere P, Kiemeneij F et al. A comparison of balloon-expandable stent implantation with balloon angioplasty in patients with coronary artery disease. Benestent Study Group. N Engl J Med 1994; 331: 489–95

5. Serruys PW, van Hout B, Bonnier H et al. Randomised comparison of implantation of heparin-coated stents with balloon angioplasty in selected patients with coronary artery disease (Benestent II). Lancet 1998; 352: 673–81

6. Cohen DJ, Taira DA, Berezin R et al. Cost-effectiveness of coronary stenting in acute myocardial infarction: results from the stent primary angioplasty in myocardial infarction (stent-PAMI) trial. Circulation 2001; 104: 3039–45

7. Greenberg D, Bakhai A, Cohen DJ. Can we afford to eliminate restenosis? Can we afford not to? J Am Coll Cardiol 2004; 43: 513–18

8. Greenberg D, Cohen DJ. Examining the economic impact of restenosis: implications for the cost-effectiveness of an antiproliferative stent. Z Kardiol 2002; 91 (Suppl 3): 137–43

9. Cutlip DE, Chauhan MS, Baim DS et al. Clinical restenosis after coronary stenting: perspectives from multicenter clinical trials. J Am Coll Cardiol 2002; 40: 2082–89

10. Hodgson JM, Bottner RK, Klein LW et al. Drug-eluting stent task force: final report and recommendations of the working committees on cost-effectiveness/economics, access to care, and medicolegal issues. Catheter Cardiovasc Interv 2004; 62: 1–17

11. The Bypass Angioplasty Revascularization Investigation (BARI) Investigators. Comparison of coronary bypass surgery with angioplasty in patients with multivessel disease. N Engl J Med 1996; 335: 217–25

12. Legrand VM, Serruys PW, Unger F et al. Three-year outcome after coronary stenting versus bypass surgery for the treatment of multivessel disease. Circulation 2004; 109: 1114–20

13. Ferreira AC, Peter AA, Salerno TA et al. Clinical impact of drug-eluting stents in changing referral practices for coronary surgical revascularization in a tertiary care center. Ann Thorac Surg 2003; 75: 485–89

14. Clark MA. Drug-eluting stent adoption and hospital finances: modeling the impact. Cath Lab Digest 2003; 107: 3008–11

15. Chaitman BR, Fisher LD, Bourassa MG et al. Effect of coronary bypass surgery on survival patterns in subsets of patients with left main coronary artery disease. Report of the Collaborative Study in Coronary Artery Surgery (CASS). Am J Cardiol 1981; 48: 765–77

16. Lemos PA, Serruys PW, Sousa JE. Drug-eluting stents: cost versus clinical benefit. Circulation 2003; 107: 3003–3007

17. Hodgson JM, King SB 3rd, Feldman T et al. SCAI statement on drug-eluting stents: practice and health care delivery implications. Catheter Cardiovasc Interv 2003; 58: 397–99

# 14. THE FUTURE OF DRUG-ELUTING STENTS

## Christopher J White

## The impact of drug-eluting stents on clinical practices

There is no question that the superior efficacy and excellent safety data of drug-eluting stents (DES) compared to bare metal stents (BMS) offer a major advance in percutaneous revascularization therapy in selected patients. Single digit restenosis rates argue for a broad implementation of this technology, which is currently outside the scope of the pivotal trials and FDA approval of these devices. Why shouldn't everyone who needs a stent have DES implanted? The major limiting factor is cost. Assessing the relative cost-benefit for each patient will be a major task facing interventional cardiologists. As newer stents appear, perhaps the unit price will fall, allowing a broader application of this technology.

When considering cost-benefit, there are multiple perspectives to be considered. The first and most important is the patient's perspective. Certainly patients prefer lower restenosis rates, which means that fewer procedures are required for percutaneous revascularization. Is there a cost at which patients would prefer a BMS? A group of patients were surveyed regarding their willingness to pay out of pocket ($100 to $5000) for a stent with a 10% restenosis rate versus a no-cost-to-them stent with a 30% restenosis rate. The median willingness to pay out of pocket for the lower restenosis rate was $1040, which translates into $5200 per restenosis event prevented.

There are several areas in which DES may have a negative impact on the overall practice of cardiovascular medicine. The transition from predominantly surgical coronary revascularization to catheter-based percutaneous procedures will mean that hospitals will perform fewer coronary bypass procedures, one of their most profitable procedures (Figure 14.1). This loss of hospital surgical revenue is exacerbated by decreasing profit margins from the catheterization laboratory caused by the incremental cost of DES. Unrestrained DES use will have a negative impact on our healthcare system, one that cannot be sustained without alternative pricing or additional private or government funding.

There is also a human resource issue to be considered. It is likely that too many cardiac surgeons have been trained for the number of heart surgeries that need to be performed, and at the same time we have trained too few cardiologists.[1] As the revascularization equation is pushed farther to the percutaneous side, the need to retrain heart surgeons as interventionalists will need to be seriously considered.

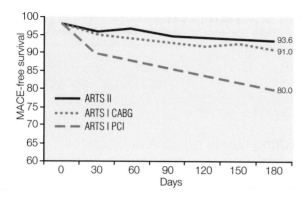

**Figure 14.1:** Adverse event-free survival for drug-eluting stents (ARTS II) is very similar to historical coronary artery bypass graft controls and superior to historical percutaneous coronary interventions. MACE, major adverse cardiac event.

## The future of drug-eluting stents

The future of DES is very bright (Box 14.1). The development of newer agents, newer delivery platforms, and broader applications will further benefit our patients and hopefully contain costs. The most serious limitation interventionalists face is the possibility of 'rationing' this expensive technology. Another limitation of the current DES systems is their inability to be delivered in a minority of cases. Trackability and deliverability of these devices should be a major focus for improvement.

**Box 14.1. Impact of drug-eluting stent technology**

- Concern over stent durability has been removed
- New directions for intervention away from restenosis:
  - percutaneous valve development
  - bifurcation technology
  - chronic total occlusion technology
- Drives physician specialty choices away from surgery
- More patients will benefit from revascularization

More data are required regarding the application of DES in more complex lesions subsets, the development of bifurcation stents, and the use of DES with adjunctive devices such as atheroablative devices (Box 14.2). Lesion subsets such as diffuse small vessel (<2.5 mm) disease, distal left main lesions, and vein graft disease remain significant challenges that are yet to be solved.

**Box 14.2. Unapproved indications for drug-eluting stents**

- Full metal jacket stent placement
- Chronic total occlusions
- Bifurcation lesions
- Left main stenosis
- Multivessel coronary disease
- In-stent restenosis
- Acute myocardial infarction

## Reference

1.  Fye WB. Introduction: the origins and implications of a growing shortage of cardiologists. J Am Coll Cardiol 2004; 44(2): 221–32

# INDEX